D1086574

STOPPING SCOLIOSIS

STOPPING SCOLIOSIS

The Complete Guide to Diagnosis and Treatment

Nancy Schommer

AVERY PUBLISHING GROUP INC.
Garden City Park, New York

The ideas, procedures, and suggestions in this book are not intended as a substitute for consulting with your physician. Proper treatment of scoliosis requires a doctor's supervision.

Cover Designers: Janine Eisner-Wall and Rudy Shur
Cover Photo Credit: SuperStock
In-House Editors: Carolyn Sofia, Marie Caratozzolo, and Elaine Will Sparber
Typesetters: Coghill Typesetting Company, Richmond, Virginia

Library of Congress Cataloging-in-Publication Data

Schommer, Nancy
    Stopping scoliosis: the complete guide to diagnosis and treatment/ Nancy Schommer.
      p. cm.
    Includes bibliographical references and index.
    ISBN 0-89529-466-4
    1. Scoliosis—Popular works. I. Title.
    RD771.S3S24 1991
    617.3'75—dc20   90-28147
                                              CIP

Printed in the United States of America

10 9 8 7 6 5 4 3

Contents

This book is dedicated to Laura Gowen,
her staff, and all the volunteers
of the National Scoliosis Foundation

Acknowledgments

I wish to thank the following individuals and organizations (listed alphabetically) who assisted me in the preparation of *Stopping Scoliosis:* Ben Allen, Jr.; the American Academy of Orthopedic Surgeons; Fred Barge; David Bradford; John C. Brown; William Bunnell; Joseph Dutkowsky; John Emans; Kurt Enslein; Laura Gowen and the staff of the National Scoliosis Foundation; Linda Hacker; Richard Herman; Neil Kahanovitz; Hugo Keim; Howard King; David Levine; John Lonstein; Alf Nachemson; Theodore Oegema; James Ogilvie; William Opsahl; Frank Rand; Thomas Renshaw; Robert Rucker; the Scoliosis Association; the Scoliosis Research Society; Dar Swanson; Joseph Sweere; Ethan Tarasov; and Robert Winter.

Special thanks to David Elmore and all the scoliosis patients and their parents who shared their experiences with me.

Foreword

When *Stopping Scoliosis* was first published, *Publisher's Weekly* applauded the book as "a compassionate, informative guide to the diagnosis and treatment of curvature of the spine." *Kirkus Reviews* hailed it as "a concise, clear explanation of scoliosis and its treatments, with plenty of practical pointers and support from fellow sufferers." Those comments are as true now as they were then. I am pleased to have the opportunity to say that the revised edition of Nancy Schommer's book is, to my knowledge, the best, most comprehensive book presently available for the layperson who is dealing with this baffling disorder.

If you have been diagnosed as having scoliosis, you should find the answers you're looking for in this book. Ms. Schommer has interviewed many of the best-known orthopedic spinal specialists to get the most up-to-date information available. With her gift for translating medical jargon into readable prose, she supplies readers with important, accurate information that's easily understood. What's more, because she has had two surgeries to correct her own scoliosis, she is able to write about her subject with sensitivity and compassion: she understands what it's like to wear a brace and to undergo surgery, and shares her insights with candor, humor, and warmth.

Stopping Scoliosis is an invaluable resource for anyone dealing with this challenging, perplexing condition.

Laura B. Gowen
President
National Scoliosis Foundation

Introduction

I see her every morning when I buy my cup of coffee at a bustling New York deli near my office. She darts back and forth behind the counter, quickly jotting down orders and stuffing bagels into white paper sacks. I watch her every move.

Perhaps seventeen, she reminds me of myself when I was that age: quick birdlike movements; sarcastic, rapid-fire banter—and a petite, wiry body that is beginning to show signs of scoliosis.

She's just as clever as I was nearly twenty years ago, but she's invented her own special way of hiding it. The preppy-looking sweater draped about her shoulders provides near-perfect camouflage. So does the smock that billows over her uniform. But every time she bends to reach into the glass case filled with pastries, I can see that her body has begun to betray her. The gnarled spine gives her secret away.

I see her every morning and the same thoughts race through my mind. Surely she must know she has scoliosis—curvature of the spine. Surely she can't ignore that twisted torso, those crooked shoulders. Surely a parent or a friend has tried to coax her into seeing a doctor about it. Then it hits me: maybe she's too proud—or scared—to admit that something's wrong. Maybe she's convinced herself that nothing can be done.

I'll probably never know the truth. I know I can't just walk up and confront her—she looks too cocky, too much like me, to accept that sort of approach. Maybe one of these days, when she's not so busy, I'll con her into having a cup of coffee with me so that I can at least tell her a story. Maybe parts of it will sound familiar to her.

Sweat trickled down the sides of my face as I spun the dial on the combination lock that secured my gym locker. As I fumbled to open it, the girl next to me pulled off one of her tennis shoes and slam-dunked it into the towel bin.

"That woman is a real sadist!" she shrieked. "Did you see who I got stuck with today? Jeez, what a pizza face!"

I chuckled, but knew just how she felt. This was the most dreaded semester in all of tenth grade—endless weeks of "modern dance," during which we spent an hour a day stumbling around the gym floor in the awkward grasps of pimply-faced boys.

"Yeah, well, did you see my partner?" I asked. "He's only about a foot shorter than me, and I swear he kept trying to look down my shirt. What a creep! Thank God I had my bra on."

"Bra? You call that 'trainer' a bra?" she teased. "Face it, Schommer, you're a plank."

My breasts were in training all right, but I thought they showed a lot of promise. In no time at all, I figured, I'd be graduating to one with real cups—the push-up kind that were guaranteed to "lift and separate." All I needed was a little more time to grow. . . .

The locker room echoed with the hoots and hollers of my classmates as we got undressed and prepared to hit the showers. I quickly wriggled out of my gym suit, wrapped a tiny white towel around me, and—quite cleverly, I thought—managed to undo my bra with one hand, slide it down the front of my body, yank it out from beneath the towel, and toss it into my locker, all in one fast, fluid movement. I sat down on the bench, slipped out of my panties, and with one foot flicked them into my gym bag. We had all become masters of deception when it came to undressing in front of one another, but I felt I had the routine down to a science.

"Schommer, what on earth are you doing? What are you trying to hide?" My sadistic gym teacher's voice bounced off the wall behind me. I clutched my towel and crossed my legs as I watched her walk toward me. She was, with her short-cropped hair, squat neck, and thick legs, what we called a real jock.

"Get rid of that towel and get into the shower," she barked.

"What do you mean?" My voice squeaked out the words.

"You heard me. We do not take our towels into the shower. I told you that weeks ago. Honestly, you girls and your modesty! Now ditch that towel and start lathering up!"

Amid all the mumbling and grumbling—none of us liked the new "no-towel" rule—I reluctantly dropped the towel, turned around, and tiptoed quickly across the cold granite floor, my arms flanked across my breasts. She was watching every move I made, and seemed genuinely pleased at my embarrassment.

"Wait a minute, Schommer. Come back here."

I fully expected a loud lecture and imagined that the girls would crowd around me while the old crone held me up to ridicule. But instead she gently took my arm, led me to a secluded area beyond earshot of my classmates, and handed me a towel. Shivering, I grabbed it and held it close.

"Stand up straight for a moment, would you, Nancy?" Her voice was so soft and gentle I couldn't believe this was the same woman who, moments ago, had tried to make a fool of me.

"What do you mean?" I asked. "I am standing up straight." Her eyes narrowed to slits; she was studying every inch of my body.

"Would you mind turning your back to me?" she asked. Oh, come on, I thought, you're just trying to torment me. Can't you see this towel isn't big enough to cover my behind? Slowly I pivoted and faced the wall.

"Do you have any back pain at all?" she asked.

"Nope. Why? What do you see?"

She put her hands on my waist and pushed in on each side.

"Can you feel that?"

"Feel what? Your hands are cold." My heart was racing now.

"Let's go over to the mirror for a moment," she said as she led me toward the bathrooms. Gently she pulled the towel to one side. "Now, do you see how one hip looks higher than the other? Can you see that little indentation on the left side of your waist?"

"No, I don't see anything," I said. "Can we just stop doing this now?"

"Okay. I'm sorry if I've embarrassed you. But I think you may have a slight curvature of the spine. That would account for your hips looking uneven. Have you ever seen a doctor about it?"

"I just had a complete physical and I checked out okay. My doctor's a really terrific guy. He'd have said something." Actually, it had been nearly a year since I'd had my last physical exam, but I wasn't up to quibbling about details. Besides, I felt just fine.

"Well, maybe it's nothing," she said. "But I think it's something you ought to watch."

"Yeah, I'll watch it," I said angrily. "I'll watch it every day and let you know what happens."

During the next several months, I did everything I could to avoid thinking about my spine. But all around me there were clues that pointed to one disturbing fact: my "slight curvature" was getting progressively worse.

Although I was just a budding clarinetist, I had set for myself the goal of winning first chair in the senior high band by the end of the year. Each day after school I locked myself in the bathroom— the only place in the house with decent acoustics where a person could have a little privacy—and blew on the old licorice stick until my cheeks hurt. My back hurt, too, but because I was spending so many hours hunched over my music book, I chalked up the slight tingling sensation and dull ache at the base of my spine to tension. Anybody's back would hurt under those conditions, right?

Faster and faster my fingers could fly over the keys and stops until finally, with almost no effort at all, I could toot my way through *Eine Kleine Nachtmusik* without having to glance at the sheet music. I thought I was pretty hot stuff and figured I now had a strong chance of beating out the competition. And even though the pains in my back were getting worse, I convinced myself they were the result of long hours of practice; perhaps pain was just the price I had to pay to reach my goal!

Chair placement day finally arrived. I squirmed in my seat, trying to get into a comfortable position. But no matter which way I turned, my back still ached, and now it felt as if sharp fingers were pinching my shoulder blades. I arched my back to try to relieve some of the pressure and found that the straighter I sat, the better I felt. But I also discovered that unless I consciously sat erect, my body just naturally slouched; it almost seemed as if my torso curved slightly to the left. Pooh! It's just your imagination, I told myself. Quit thinking about it! Concentrate on the music! As I leaned forward for one final pain-relieving stretch, I heard the dreaded words: "Nancy Schommer, you're next." Oh God, this was it!

I felt as if I was walking in slow motion as I made my way to center stage. All eyes were upon me, and I believed that each person in the room was scrutinizing my every move. Did my hair look all right? Would anyone notice my bust looked a little bigger today? (A lot of my friends wore "falsies," pointy foam rubber cups that you placed inside your bra, but I thought they looked phony, so instead I stuffed cotton balls in my bra. They began to itch now, and I regretted the deception.) Why had I worn that stupid red belt? It didn't really match my sweater, and it didn't fit that great either. It was digging into my side. But before I had a chance to try and loosen it, Mr. Snow, the band director, began his familiar chant.

"One, two, three, four, and . . ." I gulped in as much air as I could, pursed my lips around the mouthpiece, and pushed out a steady stream of air. Cautiously I tongued the first nine notes. Perfect! I was on my way!

Midway through the toughest passage of the Romanze, the tingling feeling in my back returned. As my fingers flew over the keys, I tried arching my back a little, but even that didn't relieve the sensation. I knew I was in trouble—I was having difficulty concentrating on the music—and feared that I'd have to stop to rest. Luckily, Mr. Snow suddenly waved his hand, smiled, and said that was all he needed to hear. Exhausted but happy, I returned to my seat and yanked off the belt. What a relief it was just to sit down!

I won first chair, but victory was not as sweet as I thought it would be. To keep up with the increasingly difficult music, I had to put in more hours of practice each day. As a result, my back hurt more than ever. But worse than that, the little indentation at my waist seemed to be getting bigger.

One morning, I marched straight into the bathroom, locked the door, took off all my clothes, and stood directly in front of the full-length mirror.

Head up, shoulders back, feet planted firmly on the floor, I studied every contour and ripple. I rested my hands on my hips and pushed inward. Yes, there did seem to be a slight indentation on the left side of my waist. And yes, my right hip did seem to be tilted slightly higher than the left. But the difference was so minute, I had to keep looking again and again. One moment it seemed higher; the next it seemed level with the other one. Now I was getting confused. Was there really something wrong, or was I imagining things? Maybe the little dent marked the beginning of a womanly waistline. But then why wasn't there another one on the other side? And what about the hip? What would explain its asymmetry? My thoughts drifted back to the locker room. "Slight curvature of the *spine*," the gym teacher had said. As I scrutinized my body, her comment made no sense at all. What could a slight curvature of the spine have to do with my hips?

I shifted my weight from one foot to the other, watching carefully the effect this had on my body. When I raised my left foot off the floor, my hips leveled off. After a few minutes of repeating this little soft-shoe routine, the idea finally hit me: one leg was shorter than the other. That was the problem! But how to solve it?

Half an hour later I was sitting on the edge of the toilet seat, cutting thin pieces of cardboard into small heel-shaped discs. I stacked three of them in the heel of my left shoe and looked at myself in the mirror. No discernible change in my hips. I continued inserting cardboard pieces until they reached a quarter-inch thickness. Another glance in the mirror. I seemed level at last!

I practiced walking back and forth across the room, trying to adapt to my new shoe lift, but the only way I could keep the cardboard pieces from sliding around in my shoe was by shuffling. This would never do, I thought, so I glued them together into a solid piece. Now it was easy to walk around. Better than that, the little dent at my waist seemed to have disappeared!

As you might have guessed, this gambit didn't work. What with all my activities at school, I couldn't seem to keep the lift a secret—to my horror, it slipped out of my shoe onto the floor at least once a day. And when I removed it at night and walked barefoot, my body returned to its crooked position.

Mind you, I didn't look "deformed." But even though my hips would be facing straight ahead, the upper part of my body, particularly my rib cage, seemed to be curling to the left. By this time

I wasn't feeling any kind of pain; my earlier aches, probably caused by stress or my body's reaction to my first menstrual period, had all but disappeared. Now all I felt was discomfort, for which I could get relief only by repeatedly twisting myself back to the right. Throughout my junior and senior years, I had the ominous feeling my body was fighting against some unseen force that was determined to keep me out of balance.

There was no denying it anymore. Something was wrong with my body, and I felt it had to be something more than a slight curvature of the spine. Something slight would not cause such gnarling. Whatever it was, I knew it was serious.

I was scared, but waited until after I graduated to make an appointment with a doctor. I figured if I'd gone this long, certainly a few more months couldn't hurt.

He poked at me, ran his fingers up and down my back, and told me that I had a spinal curvature. I was fully expecting that he'd prescribe a bunch of exercises, maybe even a new type of heel lift. Instead, he told me I'd have to wear a back brace for a year. That would keep the curve from getting worse, he said. And he assured me it wouldn't be nearly as bad as I thought.

The contraption I wore for the next twelve months was the closest thing to an eighteenth-century corset that I'd ever seen. It laced up the front, wound tightly around my body so that I could hardly breathe, and had two metal bars that jutted out from the back and stopped about an inch above my shoulder blades. At the top of these bars thick straps of nylon were attached; I'd pull them over my shoulders and attach them to little belt buckles that held them—and me—in place. Once rigged up, I felt I was in a strait-jacket.

Unfortunately, this "back brace" (which I have since learned was intended for people suffering from low back pain, not scoliosis) did not fix my curvature. At the end of my year of confinement, at the age of eighteen, I was more gnarled than ever. I was also angry; I had spent a year looking like a freak, and for what? Now I looked worse! I kept my wrath to myself, though; I didn't have the guts to confront this man who, like many doctors in the 1960s, was probably unaware of, or at least unschooled in, the complex disorder known as scoliosis.

I didn't have to wait long to get my own firsthand lessons about the sinister spinal deformity called scoliosis. In fact, six months later, I heard the word officially for the first time, during a physical exam that was required by the University of Minnesota for all entering freshmen. The doctor took one look at me, asked me to bend over, then shook his head.

"Well, you certainly have a case of scoliosis," he said, peering over the horn-rimmed glasses that perched on the end of his nose. "Why'd you wait so long to see a doctor?"

I was sure the doctor wouldn't want to hear the saga of how, despite all the clues I'd been given along the way, I chose to ignore my "slight" curvature of the spine. Besides, I just wanted to get on with it. What did it mean that I had scoliosis?

Before I got my answer, the doctor sent me over to an on-campus orthopedic center that specialized in the diagnosis and treatment of the disorder. There I had a series of X rays taken and met Dr. David S. Bradford, one of the leading scoliosis specialists in the country. He, too, was nonplussed that I had blithely disregarded my curvature, which now twisted within my body at more than 40 degrees. But instead of blaming me, he addressed himself to the task of explaining scoliosis to me.

Unfortunately, his medical lexicon—words such as "lateral curvature," "vertebral rotation," "skeletal maturity," and "Cobb angle"—only served to baffle me. He did, however, utter one word that I had no trouble deciphering: "surgery."

I can think of no other moment in my life when I was as frightened or as dazed. In fact, I can hardly recall what Dr. Bradford and I talked about after he said the magic word. But that's where the haziness ends. My memories of the two spine surgeries I would eventually undergo to correct my scoliosis are as vivid as any I have tucked away.

Those surgeries, each done for different reasons, were highly successful. Indeed, I have no regrets whatsoever about twice having been beneath Dr. Bradford's experienced scalpel. Today my posture is the envy of my peers, and I feel terrific. But let's not let a little healthy body worship skew the facts. Because of ignorance, pride, and fear, my family and I allowed my scoliosis to reach a point where it took a total of eight hours on an operating table, sixteen months in a plaster body cast, and untold hours of anxiety to straighten it out. Worse than all that, the entire ordeal probably could have been avoided!

1

What Is Scoliosis?

The more you know about scoliosis, and the sooner you know it, the more likely you are to stop it from progressing. If you've picked up this book because you think you have scoliosis—or know someone who may have it—you've taken the first important step toward conquering it. So let's begin by taking a look at a normal spine and learning how, through sometimes mysterious forces of nature, this marvelous architectural foundation of the human body follows a crooked path called scoliosis.

THE NORMAL SPINE

Of the more than two hundred bones that make up the entire human skeleton, perhaps the most gracefully shaped and intricately formed structure is the *spine.* Although people often like to refer to it as the *spinal column* or *backbone,* both these terms can be misleading because they give us the impression that we're speaking about one long, solid mass of bone. But if that were true, you'd never be able to nod your head up and down while you said "yes" when someone asked you for a date, nor could you shake it from side to side when you pleaded with a police officer, "No, honest, Officer, I wasn't speeding." Furthermore, you wouldn't be able to arch your back during an exam to get a little relief from the tension, and it would be impossible for you to bend over and pet your dog. Indeed, if our spines were solid structures, we'd go through life looking like rigidly constructed robots.

But thanks to the architectural talents of Mother Nature, our spines consist of approximately thirty-two individual bones in young children and twenty-six or more in adults, each slightly different, that are stacked one upon another beginning at the top of the neck and ending in the neighborhood of the rump. Each bone is called a *vertebra* (from the Latin, derived from the verb "to turn"), and several of these bones together are called *vertebrae*. The spine is sometimes referred to as the *vertebral column*.

UNDERSTANDING THE VERTEBRAE

If you run your fingers down the middle of your back, you'll feel a series of bumps or knobs; each one represents one part of a single vertebra. Now imagine that you have removed one vertebra from this mid-back area and are holding it in your hand so that the bump you felt is closest to your wrist. This is the position represented in Figure 1.1, which gives you a clear "aerial" view, as if you were looking down through your body at an individual vertebra.

Most of your vertebrae, like the one pictured, have three bony protrusions. The one that you feel as you run your fingers down your back is called the *spinous process*. On each side of this bony structure is a *transverse* ("sideways") *process;* in the thoracic, or middle, area of your back, these protrusions connect to your ribs.

In the center of a vertebra there is an area called the *vertebral, or neural, canal.* It surrounds your spinal cord, which sends messages from your brain to all other parts of your body and is protected by the bone of the spine.

In front of the neural canal you'll find the body of the vertebra, the solid, cylindrical element that most of us visualize when we think about the spine.

THE VERTEBRAL GROUPS

To understand more about how the spine is constructed, it's helpful to look at the various groups of vertebrae and to learn the special names of each one.

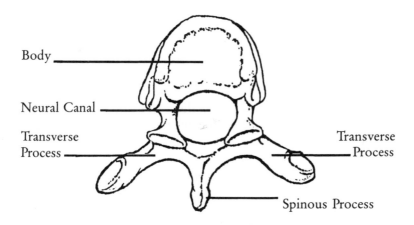

Body

Neural Canal

Transverse Process

Transverse Process

Spinous Process

Figure 1.1. The spine consists of individual bones called vertebrae. The spinous process of this thoracic vertebra is one of the bumps you feel when you run your fingers down the middle of your back.

Imagine that you have drawn a horizontal line extending from the bottom of one ear lobe to the other. At the center of this line, inside your skull, is the first of the seven *cervical vertebrae* ("cervical" derives from the Latin word meaning "neck"). The uppermost vertebra is called the *atlas,* named after the giant in Greek mythology who held the heavens on his shoulders. Just beneath the atlas lies the second cervical vertebra; it's appropriately called the *axis,* because it is this vertebra that allows us to move our head in a twisting motion. Beneath these are stacked five more vertebrae. They don't have special names, but people in the medical profession will often refer to them as C3, C4, C5, and so on.

The next group is comprised of the *thoracic vertebrae* ("thoracic" is from the Greek word for "chest"). Twelve in all, these important vertebrae not only give you support when you lean against the back of a chair, but are the structures to which your twelve pairs of ribs are attached.

If you put your hands around your waistline and slide your thumbs toward the center of your back, you will be touching the first vertebra in the *lumbar* (from the Latin for "loin") group. The five vertebrae in this area hold up the weight of most of your upper body. As a result, they are the largest vertebrae of the spinal column. Without the lumbar vertebrae we would not be able to bend over at the waist. (See Figure 1.2.)

Now move your hand to about the middle of your rump. What you'll feel is the *sacrum* (from the Latin word for "sacred"). At birth this area is made up of five tiny vertebrae. As the body grows, however, they fuse together into a solid mass of bone. The sacrum, the hipbones (or pelvic girdle), and the coccyx (see the next paragraph) are joined together to form the pelvis; the sacrum is the main support of this structure.

If you plop down on a chair, you'll be sitting on the triangular structure (made up of three tiny vertebrae, sometimes fused in the adult human being) called the *coccyx*, the lowest portion of the spine. Sometimes referred to as our "tail," the coccyx is so named because it somewhat resembles the beak of a bird (in Latin, *coccyx* means "cuckoo").

The spine is far more than just an intricate structure made up of vertebrae. From the axis to the sacrum, each vertebra is connected to the next vertebra by ligaments and muscles designed to help us bend easily. In addition, wedged between each pair of adjacent vertebrae is a rubbery, cylindrical structure called a *disc*. Made of fibrous tissue or gristle that surrounds a pulpy nucleus, the discs absorb the shocks that occur each time we walk, jump, run, or bend in any number of directions.

THE SHAPE OF THE SPINE

When you look at a person with a normal spine, viewing him or her from the side, you see that, even though he may have great posture, his back is anything but straight.

From the atlas to about the seventh cervical vertebra, the spine will curve slightly forward, then slope gently backward through the thoracic, or chest, area, then forward again in the lumbar area toward the sacrum. All normal spines have this gentle, S-shaped curve, but we're rarely aware of it, because a normal spine, when viewed from the front or back, appears to be perfectly straight. (When the spine curves abnormally toward the front or back, the result, in the upper back, is called *kyphosis*—"roundback"—or, in the lower back, *lordosis*—"swayback." These, too, are spinal deformities, but they are not scoliosis.)

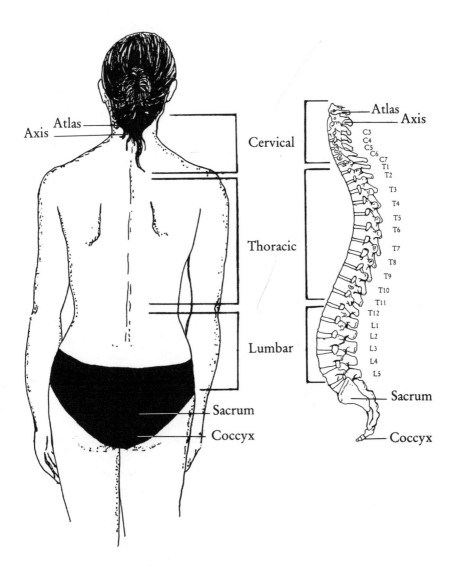

Figure 1.2. The vertebrae of the spine are named according to their position within the body. For example, the bones in the neck are called cervical vertebrae; those in the lower back are called lumbar vertebrae. Named and numbered according to location, the first thoracic vertebra is T1, the second T2, and so on.

When someone's spine begins to show signs of curving from side to side, known as a *lateral curve,* we begin to suspect that person has scoliosis. But does that mean that anyone with a side-to-side curvature of the spine has scoliosis? Well, consider the thought-provoking remarks of Dr. Robert Dickson, professor and head of Orthopaedic Surgery at St. James University Hospital, Leeds, England:

> If a scoliosis surgeon was presented with a spinal X ray and a protractor [a device for measuring the size of a curve], he could probably find a scoliosis somewhere in the spine, albeit of small magnitude. There seems to be no inherent reason why a spine consisting of [many] vertebrae piled on top of each other, separated by gristle and held up by guy ropes, growing in three dimensions simultaneously for at least fifteen years in girls and seventeen in boys, should actually *ever* be straight, and in all probability it is not.

Perhaps, then, most of us have a "touch" of scoliosis. But what's important is how much of a touch do you have, how is it affecting your body, and will it get worse?

WHEN A CURVE WORSENS

Although a side-to-side curve in the shape of a C or an S is the hallmark of the disorder, scoliosis is more complicated than that. In many cases, as the curve progresses—that is, increases or worsens—the spine also begins to rotate. It "curls" toward the hollow, or concave, side of the curve, and in advanced cases affecting the thoracic area, the ribs attached to the spine shift as well. The ribs on the concave side crowd together, while those on the convex side splay apart. Eventually the entire rib cage may narrow and become egg-shaped, crowding the heart and lungs and choking cardiopulmonary functions. In rare cases of scoliosis, victims can even die because their curves shut off their ability to breathe normally. (See Figure 1.3.)

"IDIOPATHIC" SCOLIOSIS

Although scoliosis can be caused by a birth defect, a severe accident, or neuromuscular disorders such as muscular dystrophy and polio, in 80 percent of all cases it occurs for no apparent reason at all. Hence doctors call these most common of all spinal curvatures *idiopathic,* meaning a disorder that has no cause. (That doesn't mean, however, that scientists aren't looking for the cause or causes of scoliosis. Chapter 5 provides an in-depth look at current theories that may one day lead to the discovery of a cure for this baffling disorder.)

Idiopathic scoliosis can begin in any of three stages of life. When it occurs from birth to three years of age, it is called *infantile idiopathic scoliosis;* this type is usually found in males. Considered a rare condition, the infantile curvature will improve on its own without treatment in nearly 95 percent of all cases. Although

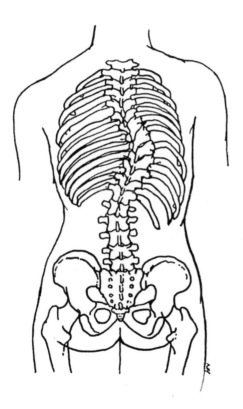

Figure 1.3. A scoliotic curve not only curves from side to side, but also rotates and causes the ribs to shift to an abnormal position. In advanced cases, rotation can cause problems in cardiopulmonary function.

scientists do not know why, infantile scoliosis is far more prevalent in Europe than in the United States.

When scoliosis strikes between the ages of four and ten, it is referred to as *juvenile idiopathic scoliosis.* This type of curve occurs in both males and females and can progress fairly rapidly as the child approaches adolescence.

The third type of scoliosis, and by far the most prevalent, is *adolescent idiopathic scoliosis.* It occurs during the growth spurt—usually between the ages of ten and thirteen—when the skeletal frame is developing most rapidly, and for unknown reasons it strikes females in seven out of every ten cases.

WHO WILL GET SCOLIOSIS?

Unfortunately, doctors cannot yet predict with great certainty who among us will get scoliosis. But if you ask orthopedists just how many youngsters in the United States are likely to develop a lateral curvature, you'll usually get this answer: one in every fifty. That sounds like a lot—until you realize that not all curves are serious or require treatment.

According to Dr. John Lonstein, an orthopedic surgeon in the Twin Cities and one of the researchers who is trying to determine the percentage of the population afflicted with scoliosis, the best way to understand the prevalence of the disorder is to convert that estimate of one in every fifty by using proportionately higher figures. Thus we may say that twenty out of every one thousand youngsters will develop a lateral curvature. "Out of this twenty," says Dr. Lonstein, "fifteen youngsters will develop curves of less than 20 degrees—degrees are a measure of how much one area of the spine curves—but few of these will get worse. The remaining five of every one thousand will have curves greater than 20 degrees, but on average, only one or two of these will increase and require treatment."

CONGENITAL SCOLIOSIS

A number of patients have asked, "Can one be *born* with scoliosis?" The answer is yes, and the condition—which is far less common than the idiopathic variety—is known as congenital scoliosis. "In these cases," says Dr. Lonstein, "when the spine was developing in the early embryonic stages, there were vertebrae that did not form properly and therefore created a curve which can get worse. You may or may not notice this condition in a child; in fact, it's quite possible for someone to have congenital scoliosis which is not detected until much later in life."

It's important to note that individuals who have congenital scoliosis oftentimes will have congenital abnormalities in some other part of their bodies as well. Notes Dr. Howard King of Northwest Spine Surgeons, Seattle, Washington, "About a third of these patients will have kidney or bladder abnormalities, and roughly twenty percent of those who have congenital scoliosis of the cervical spine also will have hearing problems. Some patients also have heart conditions."

ADULT SCOLIOSIS

"Perhaps as many as two to four million adults in the United States have scoliosis," says Dr. Lonstein. "But the majority of these are people with curves under 30 degrees that are non-progressive and never need treatment." Still, it's important to know that these individuals did not suddenly develop the disorder later in life. With the exception of people who develop *degenerative scoliosis* (see below), many adults who now have scoliosis probably developed their curves in adolescence.

DEGENERATIVE SCOLIOSIS

According to Dr. King, the condition that's referred to as degenerative scoliosis "is becoming a big problem. It occurs in older people, usually after the age of fifty, for a variety of reasons: the discs wear out, or the person develops osteoporosis, a disease that's characterized by brittle and porous bones. As the population lives longer, we'll probably be seeing more of it."

TYPES OF SPINAL CURVES

Although doctors have identified nearly a dozen curve patterns, for our purposes we will look at four major types of curves that can occur.

The *right thoracic curve,* which centers itself in the chest area, is the most common of all. It usually starts at the T4, 5, or 6 thoracic vertebra and ends around T11 or 12 or L1, the first lumbar vertebra (see Figure 1.4.) Such a curve can progress rapidly and, unless treated early enough, will shift the ribs on the right, or convex, side and create a deformity that's known as a *rib hump* on the back. Not only is the hump unsightly and the cause of much psychological stress for the person who has developed it, it's also dangerous because it can squeeze the heart and lungs, causing serious cardiopulmonary problems.

The *thoracolumbar curve,* which begins in the chest area at T4,

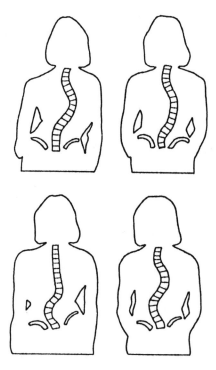

Figure 1.4.   Although doctors have identified nearly a dozen curve patterns, the most common types of curve are: right thoracic *(top left);* thoracolumbar *(top right);* lumbar *(bottom left);* and double major *(bottom right).*

5, or 6 and ends in the lower back at L2, 3, or 4, may twist to the right or the left. Although it's less deforming than a right thoracic curve, the thoracolumbar type usually creates an asymmetrical torso.

The *lumbar curve* occurs in the lower back and appears at T11 or 12 to L5. In roughly 65 percent of all cases, these curves shift to the left. A lumbar curve will twist the hips so that they appear uneven, and can cause a great deal of back pain, particularly in adults and especially in pregnant women.

The *double major curve* is the most prevalent of the S-shaped curves that occur with scoliosis. The upper part of the curve occurs in the thoracic or chest area, while the lower part affects the lumbar area. Because one curve offsets the other, the double major curve is considered more balanced and less deforming than the single C-shaped curves. But when it becomes severe, it can cause a rib hump.

HOW IS A CURVE MEASURED?

If methods for measuring curves hadn't been devised, doctors would have a hard time distinguishing between mild, moderate, and severe curves. And how confusing it would be for a patient to learn that he or she had a "really big" curve or a "pretty small" one! Thanks to the late John Cobb of the Hospital for Special Surgery in New York City, an orthopedic surgeon who developed one of the most successful methods for measuring curves, doctors now describe scoliotic curves in terms of degrees.

To measure an S-shaped double major curve, your doctor would begin by taking an X ray of your spine. Then he would start measuring the top curve, using a straightedge to draw one horizontal line just beneath the highest vertebra involved in the curve, and another just above the lowest curving vertebra. From these he would draw perpendicular lines that eventually intersect to form an angle. That angle would be measured and referred to in degrees. He would then repeat these steps to measure the bottom curve. As you can see in Figure 1.5, the Cobb angle of both curves is 65 degrees.

Because scoliotic curves often rotate as well as curve from side to side, doctors have developed a method for measuring the amount

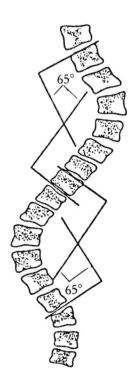

Figure 1.5. To determine how many degrees a spine is curving, most doctors use the Cobb angle of measurement. Each curve of this double major curve has a Cobb angle of 65 degrees.

of spinal rotation. As you can see in Figure 1.6, a line is drawn on an X ray in the center of each vertebra involved in the curve. When rotation is present, the oval indentations (called *pedicles*) on each vertebra shift progressively closer to the midline. To describe the relative proximity of the pedicles to the midline, doctors will refer, for example, to a +1, +2, +3, or +4 rotation.

WHOSE CURVES MUST BE TREATED?

Let's say that you suspect you have scoliosis. You meet with an orthopedist who believes it is necessary to take X rays of your spine. After he measures the Cobb angle of your curve, then figures out how much, if any, your spine is rotating, he makes this pronouncement: "You have a right thoracic curve of 22 degrees,

+1 rotation." Okay, now you know without a doubt that you have scoliosis. So your next question is, "What should I do about it?" To your utter surprise, he replies, "Well, you may not have to do anything at all."

Nothing? Do nothing about the curve? Don't I have to wear a brace or have surgery?

The answer to your questions will depend, in part, upon the maturity of your bones, or "bone age." Girls usually stop growing about age sixteen. Boys, a little slower in the growth department, finally reach maturity at around eighteen. But since we all grow at slightly different rates, these dates may vary. Thus, a girl who is chronologically fourteen may have already reached maturity, whereas a boy of eighteen may still be skeletally immature.

HOW BONE AGE IS DETERMINED

Your doctor may go back to that initial X ray and examine the *iliac crests* of your hips (you can feel them on either side by placing your hands just beneath your waistline). If you are skeletally immature, these crests will appear to be separated from the rest of the bony pelvic girdle; if you're mature, they will have fused together into a solid piece of bone.

Individual vertebrae can also provide clues to bone age. In

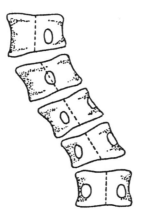

Figure 1.6. **When rotation *is* present in a curvature, the oval indentations (*pedicles*) on each vertebra will appear closer to the midline that the doctor draws on the X ray.**

immature youngsters, the *growth plates* that are located at the top and bottom of each vertebra will not have united with the vertebra. When maturation is complete, these plates (seen on an X ray) appear to be fused to each vertebra.

Your orthopedist may also take an X ray of your hand and compare it to scores of other hand X rays that have been cataloged in a special book called the *Greulich and Pyle Atlas*. Such a comparison might reveal that, say, a girl who is chronologically fourteen actually has a bone age of thirteen.

Dr. James Ogilvie, an orthopedic surgeon at the Twin Cities Scoliosis Spine Center, sums it up best: "If you take a young lady who is twelve years old with a 22-degree curvature, and she's been menstruating for two years, and is wearing a bra, and has shapely hips, you may say she's only twelve calendar years old, but when you look at her bones on X rays and see that the growth centers have all closed, you'd say she had a bone age of fifteen or sixteen. She would have already gone through the growth spurt, and we'd consider her skeletally mature. We'd continue to watch her curve, but it's unlikely that it would progress. She might not have to do a thing about her curve.

"But if you took another young lady of twelve with a 22-degree curvature, and she hadn't started menstruating yet and didn't have what we call secondary sex characteristics, we'd say this child is in a high-risk group to have a progressive curve. We'd watch her carefully, and if her curve progressed, we'd begin treatment immediately."

Predicting which curves will worsen is a laborious and often difficult task for orthopedists. But because they have amassed so much information about curves over the years, they can provide us with a few general guidelines. For example, most experts now agree that slight curves—between 10 and 15 degrees—are hardly worth worrying about, as long as they don't progress. Still, people do fret about them, according to Dr. Ogilvie. "We frequently see people who've been told by their doctors that they have scoliosis and they come to our clinic with red lights flashing and a 12-degree scoliosis, which means absolutely nothing. Not only can it not be cured, it does not need to be cured. It's like having someone come in and say, 'My doctor told me I have red hair! What do I do about it?' We don't worry about such small curves if they're not progressing—they do not have, as we doctors say, prognostic signifi-cance, which is another way of saying they're not the kinds of curves we treat."

Depending on the bone age of a person and the location and size of the curve, when it progresses to within a range of 20 to 40 degrees, doctors usually recommend that the person wear some sort of brace designed to stop the curve from progressing. But this rule of thumb holds true only for adolescents whose bones are still growing. Adult curves cannot be stopped or improved by braces.

If a youngster's curve progresses beyond 40 degrees, the best solution is surgery. "For adolescent curves of that magnitude," says Dr. Ogilvie, "surgery is the only way to stop the curve. With adults, we'd evaluate a 40-degree or greater curve on a case-by-case basis. Some adults can live with a curve of that magnitude. Others cannot, because their curves deform them, or interfere with their heart and lungs. In these cases, we can perform surgery, often with excellent results. But if people paid a visit to a scoliosis specialist at an earlier age, in most cases surgery could be avoided."

Early detection—that's the key to preventing and arresting a curve caused by idiopathic scoliosis. In fact, according to the National Scoliosis Foundation, if all American schoolchildren were screened for scoliosis and treated if they had it, the number of adults who suffer from scoliosis deformities could be reduced by as much as 80 to 90 percent in the next generation!

Doctors and public health officials throughout the country have listened to the message and convinced twenty-one states to pass laws requiring scoliosis screening in schools—fourteen of them have done so since 1981. All other states have some sort of volun-tary program in some or all schools.

Still, there will be individuals whose curvatures will go un-noticed because they've learned to compensate for them cleverly (even without realizing it) or because, through some fluke in a school system, they're able to slip past the screening room without being checked. And there will always be adults who, because they're too ashamed of the way they look or because they're convinced nothing can be done for them, will continue to suffer needlessly from their scoliosis.

Whether you're an adolescent or an adult with scoliosis, you should know this: there are treatments available today that can stop your curve from progressing, and surgical techniques that can transform a gnarled body into one that's a delight to the eye. But in order to find out whether you can benefit from these treatments, you must first figure out whether you've got scoliosis. As you'll see in the next chapter, there are special ways of detecting the disorder—diagnostic techniques that can help save you, or someone you love, from a lifetime of deformity and pain.

2

Keeping the Odds in Your Favor

How important is early detection and treatment of scoliosis? Perhaps no one knows better than forty-three-year-old Dave Elmore, an astonishingly courageous man who has spent the better part of his life battling against a spinal curvature that reached 134 degrees! "It robbed me of twenty years of my life," he says, "stripped me of self-confidence, warped my attitude toward life—all because nothing was done about it early enough."

Although there is a bright side to Dave's story—after enduring several surgical procedures to correct his scoliosis, he is today in relatively good health and a highly successful real estate broker—one cannot ignore the fact that he, as he puts it, "paid heavy dues to get there." Indeed, if you stepped into his tiny Jasper, Indiana, office and asked him about the importance of early detection, he'd sit you down, look you straight in the eye—"not caring whether or not you could see that I still have a slight hump"—and take you back to 1959, when his troubles began.

"I was fourteen or fifteen back then, and my mom noticed that I wasn't standing straight. She thought I was slouching a lot of the time. To be honest with you, I never noticed that there was anything wrong with my back. I don't ever recall thinking, 'Gee, my back is curved.' But Mom sensed something was wrong, so she hustled me to a local physician, who did X rays, and there it was—a curvature of about 35 degrees. He said, 'Dave, there's nothing we can do for you. The bones have set in place, a brace is out of the question, and we can't operate on you. Wear loose-fitting clothing. If there's pain, take some aspirin. Mostly, just be thankful you're alive. It could be worse.' He also told me that the curve would stay right where it was—it wouldn't get better, but it wouldn't get any worse.

"I took his word as gospel. I mean, he was a Doctor with a capital D, right? So I just figured I'd have to live with it, that nothing could be done for me.

"That guy was dead wrong about my curve not getting any worse. As it progressed, I developed a hump on my back that I couldn't ignore—I'd wake up every morning and see the hump! And there was no hiding it, either. If I'd go into a clothing store and pick out a suit I liked, it would have to be altered, or else one leg would end up being longer than the other. I couldn't even wear an ordinary pair of Levi's. I'd walk down the street and hear people saying, 'Hey, look at that guy.' As a result, I became very self-conscious and introverted. I knew I was different physically, and became more and more shy. Maybe that's just part of the male ego—you want to be like the other guys, but you know you're not and it bugs you. So I dealt with it by hiding from society for twenty years!

"I had a lot of pain and it just kept on getting worse. Have you ever had someone take a pliers to your skin and pull it? That's what it felt like sometimes. It's almost like there was something in my back trying to get out. I tried everything I could think of to kill the pain. I did a lot of sleeping on the floor, and in a two-week period I took a hundred aspirin.

"Because of the pain, I lost a lot of time from work, which didn't exactly please my employer. At one point he demanded that I bring him a doctor's excuse to explain a recent absence. That, believe it or not, was how this body finally got into the right hands.

"An acquaintance whose wife had had scoliosis surgery suggested I go to St. Joseph's Hospital in Savannah, Georgia. So off I went, figuring I'd hear the same song and dance: 'Sorry, Dave, there's nothing we can do for you.'

"What the doctors said to me was almost worse than that: my scoliosis, now at 134 degrees, was killing me! It was twisting my body and squeezing my heart and lungs. My heart was enlarged, and my right lung was so deformed that my breathing capacity was about half of what it should be. That came as news to me—I hardly ever paid any attention to the fact that I was short of breath most of the time.

"I could hardly believe that all that was happening to my body. But what surprised me more was this: the doctors said they could do something about it!

"I trusted them immediately, although I know I'd have trusted the devil if he'd said something could be done. I especially liked the fact that they sat me down and explained the facts to me—they didn't sugar-coat them or beat around the bush about the risks involved. And there were plenty of risks. The surgery was going to be tricky because some of my vertebrae and ribs had grown together. I had the beginnings of arthritis as well. But mostly they were worried about the danger of respiratory failure during the operation—they said my body and organs might have trouble coping as they straightened my spine.

"My primary surgeon, Dr. Andrew Sheils, said I'd probably be in the hospital for three to six weeks and have to have maybe two or three surgical procedures performed on me, plus I'd be in a cast for perhaps six months. But it didn't turn out quite that way.

"Between January 3 and March 18 of 1983 I was in the operating room six times, and they performed seven separate surgical procedures on me. I was in the hospital for nearly two and a half months and in bed so long that it got to the point where I'd forgotten what a floor felt like!

"Dr. Sheils and his colleagues took me apart, physically and mentally, and put me back together again. And it was a pretty hairy rollercoaster ride all the way. I was scared a lot of the time, one of my legs was partially paralyzed, and I had about every complication you can think of. But all things considered, I'd do it all again. I don't remember ever feeling this good! I just wish I'd had it done a lot earlier."

Although Dave might not mention it during a conversation with you, his story does not end here. Several months after his final surgery, mustering all the strength and courage derived from his heroic fight against scoliosis, he launched a statewide campaign to mandate the early detection of scoliosis in Indiana. While he lobbied for his cause, he'd buttonhole any legislator who'd listen. "I'd tell them, 'Hey, look, it's statutory that all schoolchildren be immunized against measles or polio because those diseases are life-threatening. So why not scoliosis? It's life-threatening, too!' "

After one thwarted attempt to pass a bill that would mandate school screening, Dave consulted with the National Scoliosis Foundation and, with NSF's advice, tried again. At the February 7, 1984, session of the Indiana General Assembly, he rose from his seat, walked slowly to the podium, and gave the following testimony before the members of the Senate Education Committee:

> The primary purpose of House Bill 1349 is to detect spinal deformities, such as scoliosis, early enough to allow for a less painful and less costly method of treatment, other than surgery.
>
> I know how important that is because in the early part of 1983, I underwent a series of operations to improve my spinal deformity—scoliosis. The surgeries could possibly have been avoided if this state had a mandatory screening program for spinal deformities when I was an adolescent.
>
> I do not intend to dwell on my personal pain and suffering or loss of employment, but rather on the financial impact my spinal deformity has had on the federal government, the state of Indiana, and my former employer's insurance company.
>
> Since the fall of 1982, I have been an unproductive citizen of this state and this country. Through federal programs such as Social Security Disability and subsidized housing, my deformity has cost the federal government approximately $8,180. I have also received assistance from the state of Indiana through Rehabilitation Services and other programs in excess of $7,735. The cost of my hospitalization and surgeons' fees has been in excess of $37,000—80 percent of which was paid by my former employer's insurance company. To date, the total cost of my spinal deformity, idiopathic scoliosis, has cost society in excess of $52,915. This total does not reflect lost federal or state tax revenues.
>
> It is not much to ask that school nurses and physical

education teachers know their students physically, as well as classroom teachers know their students academically. Anyone who teaches health and physical education is part of the overall "health delivery system" of this country whether they realize it or not and, therefore, prevention of disabilities through screening is an activity that properly belongs to the school physical education curriculum. Screening time would take only one class period per year and would require no hiring of additional school personnel—thirty seconds per student. No instructional time would be lost.

The effectiveness of school spinal screening and early detection cannot be overstated. In states such as Delaware, Georgia, and Massachusetts, the number of youngsters coming to surgery has been dramatically reduced.

Pragmatically speaking, it is essential to identify, locate, and treat those who suffer from spinal deformities such as scoliosis, prior to skeletal maturity. Early detection and treatment by bracing gives the patient, family, and those responsible for payment, an alternate method to the costly and life-threatening alternative—surgery.

[At this point in this speech, Dave offered some financial information to support his thesis. Since he used figures that were relevant in the 1980's, I've taken the liberty of updating the information as follows:

Today, the cost of a single-stage spinal fusion surgery, including five to seven days in the hospital, can range from $12,000 to $20,000, depending on where in the country the procedure is performed. By contrast, a rigid brace costs between $1,450 and $2,000 with no time lost from school.]

Bracing is only effective prior to skeletal maturity. Bracing can prevent the deterioration of a discovered scoliotic curve in some patients. The patient is usually a candidate when he or she falls into the range of a 20- to 40-degree curve. Bracing can improve the chances of correction to the degree that surgery could be prevented.

The less dramatic, but nonetheless important, added and hidden expenses are what may be termed support systems. This includes time lost by the parent, who must care for the child who has undergone surgical correction for scoliosis, with possible loss of wages and productivity. There is time lost by the patient because he or she cannot attend school. This may add another burden and additional costs such as special tutoring services for the child. The patient could also possibly need extensive home care provided by outside nursing services.

We should not overlook the cost savings to be realized if a bill is passed. In Delaware, where the first statewide postural screening program was tested and monitored, the Scoliosis Research Society noted that the need for surgery was [nearly] eliminated. In 1977, Blue Cross of Massachusetts spent more than $2 million in hospital costs alone for scoliosis surgeries. With the cost of brace treatment only 5 percent to 10 percent of the cost of surgery, the savings potential for health costs across this state can easily be seen to be in the millions of dollars. This means savings for everyone in medical insurance programs, not just scoliosis sufferers.

Between 1981 and 1982, thirty-eight children of this state [Indiana] had spinal fusion surgery to improve their spinal deformity. Considering that each surgery alone costs $15,000, those responsible for payment—parents, insurance companies, state and federal agencies—have spent a total of $570,000. The money spent on these surgeries could have been saved if there had been an early detection program in place in all the schools. In short, those responsible for payment have been losing money because legislation has not been passed.

House Bill 1349 does not advocate any type of diagnostic treatment, but rather it should be viewed as a preventative measure that will promise all children of this state an equal opportunity to have adequate health protection for early detection of spinal deformities, while at the same time significantly reducing the cost of that care.

So convincing was Dave's testimony that later that year Indiana's House Bill 1349 passed; the legislative vote for the bill was 97 to 0 in the house and 44 to 4 in the senate. By passing the bill, Indiana became the nineteenth state to mandate school screening for scoliosis. Twenty-one states now require their public schools to screen for scoliosis. Besides Indiana, they are Alabama, Arkansas, California, Connecticut, Delaware, Florida, Georgia, Kentucky,

Maine, Maryland, Massachusetts, Nevada, New Hampshire, New Jersey, New York (except for New York City, Buffalo, and Rochester), Pennsylvania, Rhode Island, Texas, Vermont, and Washington. Most states begin screening youngsters for scoliosis in about the fifth grade.

CURVES STILL GO UNDETECTED

If you don't live in one of the states that has recognized the importance of early detection of scoliosis, there's a chance that your scoliosis, or that of a family member or friend, could go undetected. There are several reasons for this. First, many youngsters whose bodies are just beginning to develop are self-conscious. Few people—even parents—have the opportunity to catch a glimpse of teenagers when they're scantily clad or in the nude. Second, a person who has scoliosis can "compensate" for a curve or conceal it by deliberately raising a crooked shoulder or wearing bloused clothes. I know this firsthand: by the time I had made the decision to have surgery, many of my friends and co-workers were shocked to learn there was anything wrong with me. "Why on earth are you having surgery?" they asked. "We can't tell you have a curvature of the spine!"

Third, there are certain kinds of curves that are less noticeable than others. According to Dr. Ogilvie, "If you have just a single C-shaped thoracic curve, which tends to be more cosmetically devastating than an S-shaped curve, and it reached 70 degrees, you'd look crooked. Yet someone with an S curve—70 degrees right thoracic and 70 degrees left lumbar—might not look bad at all. Even a parent wouldn't be able to see much wrong. And some people happen to have more rotation to their vertebrae than others. You could find two people who both have 50-degree curves—one has a lot of rotation, which causes a very sharp rib hump and cosmetically is just awful, whereas the other person doesn't have much rotation, and, to the untrained eye, you can't tell the curve is there."

If you think you or a family member has scoliosis, there's no reason why the curve should go undetected. There are a number of

techniques available for people with no medical background whatsoever that can help them spot a curve before it's too late.

WHAT TO LOOK FOR

Let's say you have a fourteen-year-old friend who slumps a lot and
sometimes seems to be leaning to one side. Hardly a day goes by
that her parents aren't reminding her to "stand up straight!" When
she wears a dress or a skirt, her hemline often appears crooked,
leading you to believe that perhaps her parents are right—there is
something wrong with her posture. But is her problem really poor
posture? Or is it scoliosis?

To find out, you need to get a clear view of her body, which
means she should remove all clothing except her underpants. If her
hair is long, she should pin it up so that her neck is in clear view.
She should then stand with her back toward you. Her feet should
be planted firmly on the floor to ensure proper balance, and her
arms should hang loosely by her sides. Ask her to hold her head up
in a comfortable position and to look straight ahead.

Now look at her overall posture. (See Figure 2.1.) If it's normal,
you'd be able to draw an imaginary straight line from the center of
her head to the middle of her buttocks. Her shoulders would be
level, and her shoulder blades would be symmetrical as well as
being equal in prominence. Her hips would also be level and
symmetrical, and there would be an equal distance between her
arms and body. If your friend's body matches this description, it's a
safe bet her problem is posture, because she is able to straighten
herself up by standing properly. But if she has scoliosis, her
curvature will be apparent in one or more ways even when she's
standing straight.

You might, for instance, see any number of clues that point to a
curvature of the spine. If you draw that imaginary vertical line
from head to buttocks on a person who has scoliosis, the line won't
match up with either; the head seems to be shifted off to one side of
the buttocks. You may also notice that one shoulder seems higher
than the other and that the shoulder blades are uneven—one shoulder blade may appear to be jutting out farther than the other. As
you look at her hips, you may notice that one side looks bigger or
more prominent than the other, and you may see a crease at the

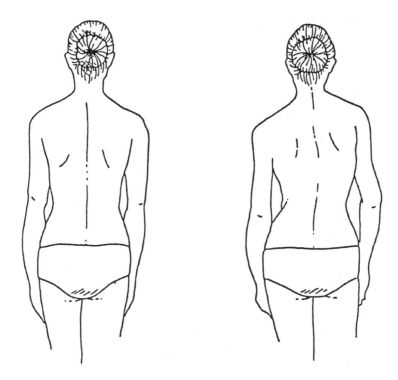

Figure 2.1.   In a normal spine *(left)*, the head is in line with the buttocks; the shoulders and hips are level and symmetrical. Scoliosis may exist *(right)* when the shoulders and hips are uneven and the waist appears creased on one side.

waistline on one side or the other—that's the little "dent" that plagued me. Moreover, the distance between her arms and her body may appear to be unequal.

In addition to examining your friend while she's standing straight, you should watch her body carefully as she participates in what's called the *forward bending test*. It's part of the screening examination used in schools across the country and can help you identify a scoliotic curve. (See Figure 2.2.)

For this exam, ask your friend to put her hands together, palms and fingers touching, and bend forward at the waist with her head down. She should be standing with her back toward you. If her spine is normal, you'll notice that both sides of her upper and lower back are symmetrical and that her hips are level and even.

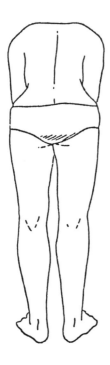 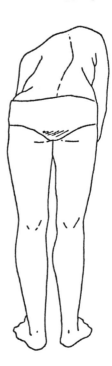

Figure 2.2.   Viewed from the rear in a forward bending test, the
normal spine *(left)* shows both sides of the upper and lower back
as symmetrical and the hips as level and even. Scoliosis may exist
(right) when the rib cage and/or lower back are asymmetrical,
with the unevenness appearing as a "hump."

If she has a spinal curvature, you may instead see that her rib
cage and/or her lower back are asymmetrical. Sometimes this
unevenness will appear as a "hump" located about the shoulder or
the lower back.

Now ask your friend to face toward you as she bends at the waist
with her hands held together as before. If her spine is normal, this
front view will reveal that both sides of her upper and lower back
are symmetrical. If not, you'll see an unequal symmetry of her
upper back or lower back, or both. (See Figure 2.3.)

IS PAIN A SYMPTOM OF SCOLIOSIS?

The answer to this question depends on whom you ask. Inter-
estingly, most doctors will tell you that scoliosis causes no pain,

particularly among adolescents. (In later life, however, adults with scoliosis can experience a great deal of pain, particularly because of breathing problems, ruptured discs, or arthritic conditions that can develop because of scoliosis.) "In fact," says Dr. John Lonstein, an orthopedic surgeon at the Minnesota Spine Center, "if a youngster with a spinal curvature complains about pain, we would look for some other cause of her curvature—a tumor or a disc injury, perhaps. If there's pain in a youngster, it's probably not idiopathic scoliosis."

In the course of my research, I've talked with many youngsters with scoliosis who claim they *did* have pain before they were treated with a brace or with surgery. Typical complaints are occa-

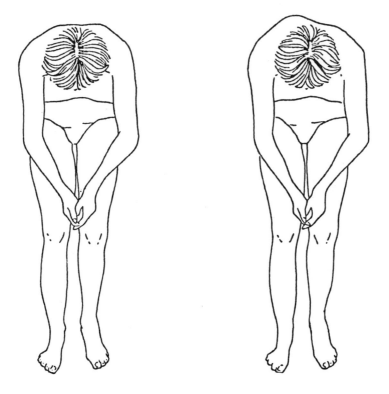

Figure 2.3. Viewed from the front in a forward bending test, the normal spine *(left)* shows both sides of the upper and lower back as symmetrical. Scoliosis may exist *(right)* if the upper back appears asymmetrical or humped.

sional numbness or tingling in the legs, aching in one or more areas of their spine, and sharp pain about the neck and shoulders.

I also know that I felt pain and tingling with my scoliosis, though the aching in my neck, shoulders, and back eventually disappeared before I had my surgery. When I've asked orthopedists about this pain, in most cases they've said it was unrelated to scoliosis.

Is that possible? Well, if you talked with Dr. David Bradford, the spine surgeon who corrected my scoliosis, and is now at the University of California in San Francisco, he'd offer a pretty strong argument in favor of that notion:

"When all these attractive kids—fourteen, sixteen, eighteen, twenty years old—come in for operations, I always ask them why they want it done. They say, 'I hurt and I want it done.' If I press them a bit and ask them why again, they'll say, 'Because it's getting worse and it bothers me. I'm active in sports and everything, but my clothes don't fit and it really hurts.' After we do the operation, when I ask them how they feel, the first thing they say is, 'Well, how do I look?'

"If I were a patient with scoliosis, I'd want that deformity fixed. And if I thought the doctor wasn't going to operate because he's not a cosmetic surgeon, he's just going to operate if there are structural problems and pain, I'd tell him it hurt, because I'd want the thing fixed."

Whether it's real or imagined, pain alone is not a reliable indicator of scoliosis. And even though the standing and forward bending tests are quite effective in helping reveal a spinal curvature, they are merely tools of detection. They cannot tell you whether or not a curve will progress, nor can they ensure that you'll get the proper treatment. Only a trained scoliosis specialist can make educated guesses about whether a curve will get worse and whether you can benefit from the many breakthroughs in nonsurgical and surgical treatment that are available today.

MONITORING YOUR CURVE

If a screening exam reveals a spinal curvature, that doesn't mean you'll be treated immediately. Most often, particularly when a curve is mild, doctors prefer to watch it for a while to see whether it progresses.

In many areas of the country, a series of X rays, taken every four to six months or so, is used to monitor a curve. Depending upon the nature and location of your curve, you may have to have as many as four X rays per visit—standing, front and back; lying down (called *supine*); and bending from side to side.

WHAT YOU NEED TO KNOW ABOUT X RAYS

Upon hearing that multiple X rays may be required to monitor a curvature, many patients become worried that they will receive "too much" radiation; they fear that their bodies will be penetrated by doses large enough to alter or destroy bodily tissue. To find out whether these fears are warranted, I recently interviewed Dr. Joseph Dutkowsky, assistant professor of Orthopedic Surgery and Pediatrics at the University of Virginia:

Dr. Dutkowsky, who first discovered X rays and why were they given that name?

The German physicist Wilhelm K. Roentgen (pronounced *rentgen*) discovered them way back in 1895. During one of his experiments, he noticed that radiation not only penetrated through the skin so he could see deeper structures like bone tissues, but it also produced phosphorescence or light. Because he didn't really know what these mysterious rays were, he named them "X" rays. Today, we know that this kind of radiation is all around us—in the atmosphere, in the ground beneath our feet, and even in our own bodies. We're all radioactive, you know. And it has nothing to do with what we eat or drink—it's just the way we're put together.

How much radiation is produced by a scoliosis X ray compared with other sources of radiation?

To answer that question, let's first talk about how radiation is measured. The standard unit of radiation is called a "rad." For measurement purposes, we usually divide a rad into thousandths, which we call "millirads." In other words, one-thousandth of a rad is one millirad. Now, to put that into perspective, consider a few figures:

- If you stayed outdoors all year round in New York City, you'd get 90 millirads of radiation.

- If you stayed in a brick building twenty-four hours a day for a year in New York City, you'd get 140 millirads.

- If you live outside the fence of a nuclear power plant, the United States government would allow you to get 125 millirads per quarter, or 500 millirads per year.

- If you have a dental X ray, you'd get 1,000 millirads.

Now, if a young girl has a scoliosis X-ray exam comprised of one PA (posterior-anterior, or back to front) X ray, plus one lateral (side-view) X ray, and assuming preventive measures have been taken to protect her breasts, her breast tissue would receive a total of 10 millirads.

Clearly, the amount of radiation from one scoliosis X ray isn't very much. But as everyone knows, X-radiation can alter tissue and destroy it. So what preventive measures do doctors use to avoid these problems?

The first preventive measure is to avoid X-radiation whenever possible. How do we do that? Well, during the course of treatment, a doctor may use a Scoliometer or other non-imaging method to monitor the patient's curve. Unfortunately, though, devices like the Scoliometer cannot give us *exact* information about a curvature; only an X ray can provide us with an extremely accurate picture of a curvature. And in certain instances—when the patient is seen for the first time and shows signs of scoliosis, or later on if his or her curve has progressed—a doctor may need to X ray the patient in order to determine the precise nature and degree of the curve. (You'll find more information about the Scoliometer and a non-imaging technique called moiré topography later in the chapter.)

In those instances when an X ray cannot be avoided, what do doctors do to lessen a patient's exposure to radiation?

First, let me tell you what doctors have done in the past several years. To begin with, they have increased and standardized the distance of the patient from the X-ray machine. Patients now stand six feet from the machine, which automatically cuts down X-radiation exposure. Secondly, they've reversed the position of the patient who must have standing X rays. Instead of having patients face the machine, which allowed X-radiation to enter sensitive breast tissue first, we now turn them around so their backs face the machine. By doing this, the spine and ribs absorb the radiation before it reaches the breasts.

What else can be done?

Doctors use a variety of lead shields that block roughly 99 percent of the radiation generated via an X-ray machine. For young girls, whose breast tissue is the most sensitive to radiation, we use breast shields. Made of lead and covered with heavy cloth, they look a lot like aprons and cover the breast area during X-radiation. When necessary, we also use lead shields that protect the female's pelvic region where the reproductive organs are located. For young boys, we use lead shields for the gonadal area. In addition, all modern X-ray machines have lead shields built right into them.

Since today's X-ray machines already contain lead shields for protection against radiation, is it necessary to use the breast and/or gonadal shields as well?

I think it's a good idea to do things twice as well as you need. By using the lead aprons for breasts and/or gonads, you're adding another measure of safety. At scoliosis clinics, using these aprons is a standard procedure.

I've heard about something called "rare earth screens." What are they and what do they do?

I'm glad you brought that up, because that's another way that we can lessen X-radiation exposure. Placed on each side of an X-ray film, rare earth screens allow more light to flash on the film to expose it. Because rare earth screens produce more light, you can use fewer X rays to get the same picture. For that reason, all scoliosis clinics today use rare earth screens.

Even with all the preventive measures now being used, particularly those that protect sensitive breast tissue, what is the risk of breast cancer in young girls who've had scoliosis X-ray exams?

We've made a lot of progress in that area, too. In 1979, Dr.

Clyde Nash did a study indicating that the typical female adolescent with scoliosis would undergo twenty-two X-ray exams during the course of treatment. Due to those X rays, he estimated the risk of breast cancer would increase 110 percent. In my most recent study, which takes into account the many preventive measures that I've already mentioned, we've found that the risk has been lowered to roughly a quarter of one percent. In other words, assuming that twenty-two radiographic examinations are performed over the course of scoliosis treatment—a far greater number of X rays than one would receive today—our findings reveal that the increased relative risk of breast cancer is roughly two breast cancers per million women examined. That's an extremely small number considering that the risk of a woman getting breast cancer in her lifetime in the United States is one out of eleven.

Even though your figures are relatively reassuring, we all want to try to protect ourselves from radiation as much as possible. Any other recommendations?

When you have to have an X ray, ask questions about the equipment and procedures. Remember, you have the right to demand any or all of the preventive measures I've mentioned. I believe that the patient's body is ultimately his or her responsibility. The more you know about the care you're getting, the more informed and comfortable you'll be—and that helps doctors do their jobs. Most, if not all, scoliosis clinics will be using the procedures I've mentioned, but it never hurts to ask questions to reassure yourself. You'll feel better about what's being done.

What about the future? Are other devices in the works?

The best "replacement" technology will probably be magnetic resonance imaging or MRI—it doesn't use any radiation at all to get a picture of the inside of the human body. Simply explained, it's a magnetic device that's used with a computer to provide exquisitely detailed, three-dimensional images. If scientists can figure out how to make it less expensive, more available, and faster at developing images, I suspect it eventually will be the ultimate tool.

TWO NEW MONITORING TECHNIQUES

Some orthopedists, such as Dr. John Emans of Children's Hospital in Boston, are trying to lessen their patients' exposure to radiation by using a technique called moiré topography.

The patient stands behind an illuminated, fine-lined grid that throws a symmetrical pattern of shadows onto the contours of the back. If the patient has scoliosis, the pattern will be asymmetrical. Dr. Emans and others who use moiré topography record these patterns with Polaroid pictures and compare the photographs taken during successive visits to detect any changes. "We're able to see pretty clearly when a curve has progressed," says Dr. Emans, "and patients don't have to worry about radiation exposure."

Another device now available for screening is called a Scoliometer. Developed by Dr. William P. Bunnell who is now at Loma Linda University Medical Center in Loma Linda, California, it is used primarily to measure the angle of rotation. It is thin and rectangular-shaped, about the size of a small envelope. A U-shaped glass tube filled with fluid has a small ball positioned in the center of it. When the doctor places this device on the back of a patient who is bending over, the ball quickly seeks the lowest point in the tube, from which the angle of rotation can be measured.

Even though the Scoliometer and moiré topography are becoming increasingly popular as effective ways of monitoring curves, orthopedists must still rely upon X rays to determine the exact nature and extent of a curve.

HOW LONG SHOULD
MONITORING CONTINUE?

Many doctors recommend that adolescents who have mild scoliotic curves need to return to the clinic for observation only every six months or so until they reach skeletal maturity. But according to Dr. Hugo Keim, an orthopedic surgeon at the New York Orthopaedic Hospital of the Columbia-Presbyterian Medical Center in New York City, "The worst advice a physician can give a patient with scoliosis is, 'As soon as you finish growing, your curve will stop.' The hundreds of adults seen each year with painful adult scoliosis attest to the fact that the disorder can progress. Scoliosis patients must have physical examinations at least biannually during their entire adult life, and if curve progression is noted, treatment must be instituted at once."

PREGNANCY AND SCOLIOSIS

In the past, many doctors believed that pregnancy would increase the risk of progression of a curve—as much as 6 to 8 degrees with each pregnancy—in a scoliotic patient after she reached skeletal maturity. Of course, that was worrisome to women with scoliosis who wanted to have children—they assumed that because they had the disorder, they would have to forego the joys of motherhood. But now, thanks to recent findings of a study undertaken by Dr. William Bunnell, scoliotic women who wish to have children have little to fear.

According to Dr. Bunnell, who completed the study while he was at the Alfred I. du Pont Institute in Wilmington, Delaware, "It was our early conclusive finding that pregnancy does not increase the risk of problems developing in patients with scoliosis. In other words, there is no increased risk that the curve will increase. In addition, there did not seem to be an increased incidence of back pain in the patients we studied. We also looked at the impact that scoliosis might have on pregnancy and delivery. Here, too, we found no increased incidence or problems including the need for a Caesarean section, or any increased problems with the children. In essence, our findings show that women should be able to look forward to normal pregnancy and delivery with no increased risk either to themselves or to their pregnancy as a result of having scoliosis."

CURVES CAN WORSEN IN ADULTHOOD

Although orthopedists cannot predict whose curves will worsen in adulthood, Dr. Keim suggests that scoliosis is most likely to progress during adult life in these sorts of patients: "Those with a strong genetic 'dose' of scoliosis; those with a curve pattern that throws the trunk out of balance, such as the thoracic, thoracolumbar, or lumbar curves; and those with extremely poor muscle tone, especially women who have become overweight and underexercised." Dr. Keim is quick to point out that "naturally not all scoliosis patients get worse as they get older, but curves in those who meet the previous criteria generally progress one to two degrees with each year of adult life."

Unless you are monitored by a specialist who knows that scoliosis can progress in adulthood, you run the risk of being told that you shouldn't be too concerned about your curve and that all will be well for the rest of your life. The remarks may be comforting at the time, but imagine how you will feel if your curve follows the same path as these patients of Dr. Keim:

> A. D. was first examined for scoliosis at age thirteen years and three months. She then had a right thoracic curve of 33 degrees from T4 to L1. A well-meaning physician advised her that this was a mild curve and told her "not to worry" about it since it would "never get worse."
>
> By age fifteen years and eight months her curve had increased to 45 degrees, but the advice was still the same. An orthopedist was consulted and also advised no treatment. This advice at first seemed correct because at age seventeen years and nine months the curve was still 45 degrees and seemed stable.
>
> However, over the next nine years she noticed gradual curve progression and increasing back pain. When I met her, she was twenty-six years and eight months old and had a 61-degree curve. She noted shortness of breath during swimming and tennis and had curtailed these activities. Feeling so much more deformed, she experienced depression, had a poor social life, and believed she had been given the wrong medical advice by her previous physicians.
>
> V. P., a twenty-one-year-old woman, had a left thoracolumbar scoliosis from T10 to L3. She was obviously fully mature and was told "not to worry" about her 20-degree curve. At age forty-two the curve had progressed only 5 degrees and she was pleased that she had no pain. She had not married and had never been pregnant.
>
> At age fifty-three the curve had progressed to 48 degrees (a 28-degree increase since age twenty-one) and she was beginning to have severe back pain and disability. She also had to give up her job as a beauty parlor operator. Surgery at that

time had to be more extensive and complicated than preventive treatment at a younger age would have been.

M. K., a very attractive young lady, was under "observation" by an orthopedist from age fourteen to twenty-eight. She had been told that her severe curves would not get worse because at age sixteen and a half she was "fully mature." She had a right thoracic scoliosis of 90 degrees from T5 to T11 and a left lumbar curve of 87 degrees from T11 to L4.

She was so concerned about health problems that she became a nurse and was examined on several occasions by orthopedists and told to "leave well enough alone." By age twenty-seven her right thoracic curve had increased to 105 degrees and the left lumbar curve also measured 105 degrees. She was having marked shortness of breath and increasing back pain.

On her own volition, she sought surgical help for her curves and had successful surgery performed with satisfactory correction—for her age.

M. G., a twenty-six-year-old librarian, was first concerned about her scoliosis at age fourteen. Her curve measured 43 degrees. She saw several orthopedists over the next six years, but was told that no further progression would occur. At age twenty-six she appeared for treatment with a curve that measured 63 degrees. She was saddened and disillusioned by the poor advice she had received. A good surgical correction was obtained at that time, but not as much as she could have had at age seventeen when her spine was more flexible and the curve less severe.

CAN EXERCISE HELP A CURVE?

Not only should you be wary of the physician who tells you "not to worry" about your curve because it won't progress into adulthood, you should also be suspicious of the doctor who recommends exercise as the sole treatment for your curvature. He is misinformed, says Dr. Ogilvie. "Voluntary exercise alone will never improve or eliminate a curve, because the brain cannot command specific paraspinal muscles [muscles next to the spine] to contract and relax. It is those muscles and surrounding tissues, when strong and healthy, that keep a spine in a straight position. When they're weak on one side or the other, the spine will bend. And even if the brain could make the right connection, who would have the discipline or stamina necessary to carry out such an exercise program?"

Although there are physicians who prescribe exercises for patients with scoliosis and who believe that daily flexes and bends can help a curvature, none of them can provide concrete evidence that exercise is an effective solution to the problem of scoliosis. "There is no real scientific evidence that exercise will affect a curve that is progressing," says Dr. Lonstein. "When studies have been done on this, where half the kids are put through really intense exercises and the other half do nothing, there's no difference between the two groups. Although we know that exercise programs are quite popular in Europe, where kids are exercising for one to two hours each day, we don't yet know whether it's making any difference. So far, there's never been any documentation of results."

Until such data exist, scoliosis specialists will continue to try to spread the word that exercise is not a cure for scoliosis. The message needs to reach adolescents and their parents, as well as medical students and residents who will become the specialists of tomorrow. Even though you'd think these highly trained individuals would get the message through the medical grapevine, often they don't, which is why there are still many physicians prescribing exercises for their scoliosis patients. Thus, experienced orthopedists like Dr. Keim have tried to make the point perfectly clear in medical textbooks such as *The Adolescent Spine.* In the second edition of this widely used reference book, he makes an extremely persuasive case against exercise. Although it is intended to be read by physicians, it will give you a good deal of "insider" information about why exercises alone should be avoided:

> One fact has been clearly shown . . . exercises never "correct scoliosis." They maintain and enhance body tone and are of value to the patient and family because they make the parents feel that they are doing something, which assuages their guilt feelings somewhat. However, do not be deluded that curve improvement could possibly be due to an hour or two of exercise which the patient may have done daily during the previous few months. The scoliotic spine is genetically programmed much like a computer to develop a specific curvature as growth progresses. This programming is determined by the genetic dose of scoliosis . . . received the mo-

ment the egg and sperm became one. The scoliotic curve that the patient will have [many] years hence can only be modified at specific times in the patient's life by either spinal bracing . . . surgery, or a combination of treatments. . . .

Sometimes we see curves vacillate back and forth until the patient is fully mature with the final end result of a very mild curve. If an exercise program had been given to these patients, there would be hundreds of enthusiastic patients and parents who would gladly sign affidavits that exercises "did the trick."

Unfortunately, we cannot yet predict which scoliosis patients will improve spontaneously and which will get worse. We need a simple test which could tell us how strong a genetic dose of scoliosis a patient has inherited. We could then advise the family that the patient will never get worse or conversely that the patient has an extremely severe form of scoliosis and should be treated in the most aggressive manner.

To sum up the indications for an exercise program, you can prescribe it if you wish, as long as you understand that exercises only treat the psyches of the parents and help the muscle coordination of certain poorly muscled children, who are overweight and underexercised.

If your doctor prescribes exercises for you, make sure that he is doing it to help you improve muscle tone. If he tells you that they alone will stop your curve, consult with another orthopedist immediately.

CAN CHIROPRACTIC HELP SCOLIOSIS?

Unlike people with arthritis, for example, individuals with scoliosis have not yet been exposed to fraudulent treatments that claim to "cure" the disorder. You won't find splashy advertisements in the *National Enquirer* touting snake oil as a panacea for scoliosis, nor will you hear rumors that a few bee stings can stop a curve. But there is a branch of the medical community involved in scoliosis care that has become the focus of much controversy, and the pivotal question of the debate is this: can chiropractors prevent or stop a curve from progressing?

As you've probably guessed, the answer you receive depends

upon whom you ask. According to one highly respected orthopedist, who asked to remain anonymous, but whose attitude reflects the opinion of many scoliosis specialists I interviewed, "We've got lots of patients who come to us from chiropractors because they've gotten nothing out of manipulation. They come to us with curves that have progressed. Still, many chiropractors contend that they can help kids with scoliosis and they offer us 'proof'—in the form of X rays, not scientific documentation—that they've done so. I can see why they think they're successful at treating scoliosis, because if they treat a hundred kids with manipulation, they're going to be 'successful' with eighty out of a hundred, because eighty out of a hundred kids are not progressive anyway. In other words, if you do chiropractic manipulation on somebody who doesn't need treatment, you're going to get a fantastic result. Therefore some chiropractors believe they can help scoliosis. But some know they cannot."

Dr. Fred Barge of the Barge Chiropractic Clinic in La Crosse, Wisconsin, is one of many chiropractors who believes that by adjusting the spine—using the hands to apply a thrust that repositions misaligned vertebrae—he can indeed correct a scoliotic curvature of the spine. Of course, Dr. Barge knows that these "dynamic thrusts" cannot benefit everyone with scoliosis, and he readily admits that "chiropractic never claims to cure any disease." Yet, based on his work with scoliosis patients throughout a career that spans thirty years, he is quite convinced that "we can reduce curves if we get to them in time."

According to Dr. Barge, when vertebrae become "subluxated"—a term used by chiropractors to describe a misalignment—the center of the discs between these vertebrae shift to one side. "Like a teeter-totter," he explains, "the fulcrum shifts and causes what we call vertebral locking. The body responds to this by forming a scoliosis, and so my job is to help free up that locking, to restore the vertebrae to their normal position." When he applies those hand thrusts (adjustments) to the patient's back over a period of time, he says, "we can achieve an improvement."

Just how often a person needs these spinal readjustments is, in Dr. Barge's opinion, "determined by the amount of benefit the person is receiving. If a young girl came to me with a curvature under 30 degrees, and she was still growing, I might have her come in for adjustments twice a week for two months, then once a week for another month. Then I'd X ray her again to see whether I was making any improvement, and if so, I'd continue adjusting the child once a week for perhaps another four to five months. I'd re-evaluate her again, have her come in every other week for a year, and when I'd achieved enough improvement, I'd recommend she have adjustments once a month indefinitely."

When a patient's curve does not respond to chiropractic treatment, Dr. Barge often refers the individual to a scoliosis specialist. "One such patient was a girl of twelve. She was at the peak of her growth spurt, wearing a brace, and her curve was 58 degrees and progressing. She came to me and cried, saying she couldn't stand the brace, so I worked with her and tried to readjust her, but the curve just kept on getting worse. I was able to reduce her lumbar curve a bit, but not the thoracic curve one iota. I referred her to an orthopedic surgeon who corrected her thoracic scoliosis through the surgical implantation of rods. In her case, neither a brace nor chiropractic treatment could help."

Despite his willingness to refer highly curved patients to specialists, Dr. Barge is not willing to go along with the opinion of many orthopedists that a curve treated chiropractically "would have gotten better by itself. Although we don't have any controlled studies to prove it, you can see the results spontaneously and objectively to prove our work."

Not all chiropractors share Dr. Barge's enthusiasm. In fact, according to Dr. Joseph Sweere, director of the Department of Occupational and Community Health at the Northwestern College of Chiropractic in Bloomington, Minnesota, "In an advanced case of scoliosis—and even a 20-degree curvature is in my opinion a significant distortion—there's little I could do to make it better."

For Dr. Sweere and other chiropractors across the country who share his view, "the primary service of a chiropractor to the children of America is early evaluation and detection of a curvature. Often, by the time scoliosis is diagnosed, it's rather late to be seeing a chiropractor. Unfortunately, because we chiropractors are often the second, third, or fourth choice in terms of doctoring, we often get patients whose curves are quite advanced. We're considered the doctors of last resort."

Although Dr. Sweere believes such patients should be referred immediately to a scoliosis specialist, he does not rule out the possibility that a chiropractor might be able to help as well. But in such cases the person would probably seek the services of a chiropractor for relief of pain.

"I've never known of a better system to help pain," he says. "It simply works, and, for pain, chiropractic can be profoundly useful for those with scoliosis. If a lady is forty years old and having a backache due to a curvature, she certainly needs a good surgical opinion and work-up—from more than one person—but there may be justification for a chiropractor to treat her as well. It may be the only relief this woman can get. In fact, I've had people come to me with 65-degree curves and I send them to the scoliosis clinic for evaluation, where the doctors say to them, 'If you can get relief from a chiropractor, then do it.' Very often orthopedists will encourage their patients to see chiropractors for pain simply because it's a practical measure. But these are orthopedists who are open-minded—they're willing to work with us to aid a common cause."

Of course, that common cause should be the early detection and prevention of scoliosis. But until chiropractors can supply us with documented, scientific evidence that spinal manipulation really can treat curvatures, their primary function should be, as Dr. Sweere and others believe, in the area of diagnosis. "What's important to know about chiropractors," says Dr. Sweere, "is that they will probably continue to be criticized for not having controlled studies and will therefore continue to lack credibility in the medical community. It should be noted, however, that we lack controlled research studies because our profession, historically, has never had any financial support with which to do the studies it so desperately wants to do. Despite the criticism, however, chiropractors are licensed and obligated to diagnose scoliosis. Many chiropractors have had special training in orthopedics and, as such, can be trusted to do it well. They know what they can and cannot do for scoliosis. Others may not have the interest or inclination to deal with this rather complex problem. If there is any question as to the qualification of the chiropractor you have consulted, it is well to contact the Board of Chiropractic Examiners in the state in which you live."

Since it's unlikely that chiropractors will amass much scientific evidence about their craft in the near future, it's probably safer to rely on the treatments for scoliosis, discussed in the following chapters, that are currently available.

3

Nonsurgical Treatments
For Use by Children Whose Curves
Range from 20 to 40 Degrees

Although patients with a curve smaller than 20 degrees sometimes require treatment, the question of whether or not to brace or perform surgery arises most often in those cases where the curve falls in the 20- to 40-degree range. (Once the spinal deviation approaches or surpasses the 50-degree point, studies show that skeletally immature patients' curves *will* progress into adulthood.) Doctors make recommendations for bracing or surgery based on a number of factors, including the size of the curvature, its location, and the skeletal maturity of the patient. This chapter surveys the major types of nonsurgical intervention prescribed for adolescents with scoliosis.

RIGID BRACING CAN STOP A CURVE

Ever since the Greek physician Hippocrates (ca. 460–377 B.C.) began studying *skoliosis* (meaning crooked), doctors have tried to straighten the curved spines of their patients by using treatments that involved the application of forces that would stretch and/or push the curving vertebrae. In most cases—at least until the twentieth century—their patients probably felt that the "treatment" was worse than having the disorder.

Centuries ago your doctor might have strapped you to a medieval-looking rack for many hours at a time over several months. Your arms and legs would have been forcibly stretched in opposite directions with an intricate system of weights, pulleys, and ropes. Or, because your physician figured that gravity played some part in pulling your spine and making your curve bigger, he might have opted for a "passive" cure—complete bed rest, for two or three years!

In time, doctors took a more sensible approach to caring for their patients; they tried to devise ways to straighten spines that would enable their patients to get up and move around. For some physicians, this meant bandaging a patient's body to splints—a rather cumbersome and uncomfortable way to keep a curvature from progressing. By the mid-1500s treatments were much more sophisticated: with the help of armorers, doctors fashioned metal corsets that were intended to hold the body straight. But these "iron maidens" probably weighed twenty to thirty pounds; under that kind of stress, patients no doubt ended up with rounded backs in addition to having scoliosis. These iron corsets eventually were replaced by ones made out of strips of leather, or by an innovative "jacket" that was molded from plaster of Paris.

Such plaster jackets represented the haute couture of braces at that time. They were relatively lightweight, were cheaper to make than the metal molds, and fit snugly to the body. It's also likely that they were more successful than their predecessors, if only because the people wearing them couldn't take them off. Of course, these plaster molds interfered with bathing and restricted the normal movements of the poor souls who were encased in them—especially those patients whose doctors, believing that more plaster meant more correction, kept on adding plaster until it covered the patient's neck and most of the head!

These plaster torture chambers provided "passive" correction: the brace did all the work to hold the body straight, and all the patient had to do was endure it. But some doctors believed their patients might do better with "active" braces—devices that forced the body to interact with the brace.

In the late 1800s physicians created a corsetlike contraption that bound the lower body in leathery material while metal bars that looked like suspenders fit over the chest and shoulders. Attached to these bars was a metal neck ring with sharp protruding buttons that fit just beneath the chin and behind the back of the neck. Unless the patient stood perfectly straight—indeed, he was forced to stretch and elongate his body—those irksome little buttons would jab fiercely into his skin. Needless to say, this brace was not too popular and probably did more harm than good.

Only within the last thirty years have doctors developed bracing techniques that are acceptable to the patients who have to wear them. And most of the credit goes to two men: Drs. Walter Blount and the late Albert Schmidt of the Medical College of Wisconsin and Milwaukee's Children's Hospital. Initially they developed a rigid support system for polio victims who'd had surgery. But today their Milwaukee brace is the standard by which all braces for scoliosis are measured. As you'll see, they incorporated some of the techniques developed by their predecessors—neck rings and metal bars, for example—but they modified them so that they're not only more comfortable than in the past, they work effectively as well. According to Dr. Lonstein, Milwaukee braces (and other rigid braces) can stop curves 80 percent to 85 percent of the time.

THE MILWAUKEE BRACE

Usually, when a youngster finds out she has to wear a Milwaukee brace, her reaction sounds something like this: "No way. It's ugly. I'm not wearing that thing." And who can blame her?

First her eyes are drawn to its largest component: the molded plastic *pelvic girdle*. (See Figure 3.1.) It looks heavy, cumbersome, and downright uncomfortable. She can't imagine how she'll be able to walk with it pushing against her abdomen, hips, and derriere. Then she wonders, "How will I bend over? Won't it jab me in the stomach? And pinch my bottom when I sit? What about my skin? After sweating in this thing all day, won't my skin become shriveled, or rot?"

Those fears seem trivial compared to what she feels when she inspects the upper portion of the brace. Nothing like a metal bar thrusting up the front of it—right between the breasts—to give one

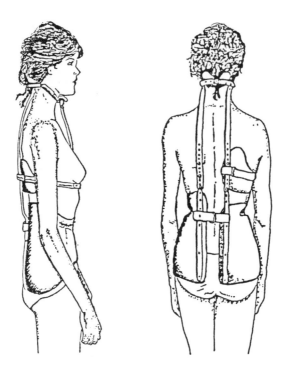

Figure 3.1. The Milwaukee brace consists of a pelvic girdle, throat mold, and various bars, straps, and pressure pads that work together to hold a curvature, that is, to try to prevent it from progressing further.

cause for alarm. "Will I have to give up wearing a bra?" she wonders.

As if that weren't bad enough, she sees that the central bar attaches to a strap that winds around around the body and is affixed to one of the metal bars in back. (Depending on the type of curvature, one's brace may contain more than one of these straps, which hold specially designed pads that support the spine in the best alignment.)

At the back of the brace, two metal bars run lengthwise and parallel over the shoulder blades. These bars rise to the back of the neck, where they converge with a *throat mold,* a sturdy piece of metal that encircles the neck like a collar or ring.

"Isn't it going to strangle me?" she asks. Then the final question: "How on earth will I ever conceal all this hardware?"

Let's face it: no one—except maybe doctors—would say that the Milwaukee brace is an attractive piece of hardware. But despite its appearance, the Milwaukee brace is a pretty amazing device—all those straps and bars, even the neck ring, are there for a specific purpose. Together, they will force your body and your spine into a straightened position while you're growing so that your curve doesn't get worse.

How It's Made

After your doctor has determined that you're a good candidate for a Milwaukee brace, she won't just pull one out of a stockroom, strap you into it, and send you home. Instead, she'll send you to an orthotist, a trained professional who will custom-make all or part of your brace, sometimes using prefabricated sections, so that it fits you perfectly and comfortably. The cost of a rigid brace ranges from $1,450 to $2,000 and should be covered by medical insurance.

The Pelvic Girdle

The structural foundation of any brace is the pelvic girdle, the molded structure that fits snugly around the waist, hips, and buttocks. Many scoliosis clinics and brace shops across the country now offer prefabricated molds that can be adjusted to fit your body. But some clinics still prefer a more traditional approach: making the molds from scratch, a procedure that involves the use of plaster.

To begin, you'll be asked to remove your clothing and put on two layers of stockinettes, or body stockings. The inner layer will protect your skin from the plaster, and the outer layer will adhere to the plaster.

You'll stand inside a special frame and rest your arms on a crossbar at shoulder level so that your elbows are parallel with the floor. Then you'll lean back on another bar just behind you and bend your knees so that your body stretches as straight as possible. Sometimes, especially if your curve is in the neck area, you may have to wear a head halter during the procedure to keep the cervical vertebrae straight. Now, to pull your body even straighter, the orthotist will cinch your waist with a strap that's attached to a lower part of the frame, and he'll adjust the strap until your waist and hips are in their proper alignment.

This "stretching" procedure may try your patience, and you may be a bit embarrassed by having to stand in such a seemingly awkward position for half an hour or so. But it's best to just grin and bear it—this is an essential part of the brace-making procedure!

Your orthotist and an assistant will dunk strips of gauzelike material into liquid plaster, then begin to wrap your body in them, from just beneath the breasts to a few inches below your hips. You'll begin to look and feel like a mummy, and as the plaster starts to harden, you'll feel a warming sensation. When the plaster finally hardens into a shell, you'll begin to feel a bit chilled, but not to worry—it's almost over!

After your orthotist takes a few measurements and makes a few adjustments, he'll remove the mold with a vibrating device. From this mold he will make another one out of plastic. This process can take anywhere from twenty-four hours to three weeks. Then he'll invite you back to try it on, at which time he'll make any adjustments that are necessary. If it's too big or small in certain areas, he'll remove it, heat it in a special oven, and compress or widen it until it fits you perfectly. If the new mold digs into your hips, waist, lower abdomen, or buttocks, he'll trim it—and smooth the edges, of course—so that it fits comfortably.

These last two steps—size adjustment and trimming—are all that's required if you're one of the many youngsters who can fit into the prefabricated type of pelvic girdle.

Once the pelvic girdle fits perfectly, the orthotist will add the metal bars: one in the front and two running parallel up the back. He does this not only to keep you as erect as possible, but also so that he has structures to which he can attach the neck ring and the straps.

Why a neck ring?

You may have the feeling that the neck ring is attached to your brace for purely sadistic reasons, but in fact it has two important functions. First, the ring attaches to and stabilizes the upright metal bars. Second, it has the ability to keep your torso balanced over your pelvis. In some cases, the neck ring may be attached temporarily to an *axillary sling* (not shown), which begins just beneath the throat mold, angles down under your armpit, and comes back up and attaches to one of the parallel bars. If you have a right thoracic curve, your upper body will tend to list to the right and the axillary sling will be placed under your left arm. Each time your body tries to lean right, the sling will pull you to the left and keep your neck in the middle of the ring. Without this sling attached, your neck would continually rub against the ring—a very uncomfortable situation! This pulling will not continue forever: after you've spent four to six months in the brace, the action of the sling will "teach" your body to balance itself automatically, and the sling can be removed.

Inside the brace

So far we have a brace that consists of a snug-fitting pelvic girdle plus metal bars—one in front and two in back—that hold the body erect. We also have a neck ring and, possibly, an axillary sling, which together keep the head and neck centered over the body and prevent them from leaning to one side or the other. All of these elements encourage you to stand up straight and elongate your spine. Shouldn't all this be enough to stop a curve from getting worse?

Unfortunately not. In order to hold a curve, a brace must also exert force against the sides of the curvature. For this reason, the Milwaukee brace also contains pressure pads that push on a curve while they interact with the forces created by the neck ring and, in some cases, the axillary sling. The result? A type of tug-of-war on the body that prevents the curve from progressing.

If you have a right thoracic curve, your spine would begin curving in the vicinity of your shoulder blades, bow out to the side in the center of your body, and curve back near your waistline. As a result, your upper body would jut out to the right, while your hips would veer toward the left. To correct this imbalance, an orthotist would place a pressure pad inside the brace on the bulging side of the curve, at a point on your rib cage that matched the apex, or top, of the curve. But he'd also have to apply a counteracting force to keep that left hip from jutting out farther. Thus, he would insert a lumbar pad inside the pelvic girdle (on the left), which would push your torso to the right. The counteracting forces of all the pressure pads, the pelvic girdle, the neck ring, and an axillary sling (if required), hold the body straight.

THE LOW-PROFILE BRACE

If you have a low curve, you'll probably be able to wear an underarm brace called the TLSO, or *thoracic-lumbar-sacral orthosis*. It's also known as an underarm brace or a "Boston bucket," named for the city where it was developed. But depending upon where you live, you may get a similar brace with a different name—the "Miami" brace, for example, or the "New York" low-profile brace. (See Figure 3.2.)

No matter what you call it, this type of rigid brace is extremely popular with patients because it's much less restrictive than a Milwaukee. The TLSO begins just beneath your armpits and under the breasts and ends near the pelvic area in the front and in the middle of your buttocks in the back. It's made of plastic—either prefabricated or custom-molded—and is generally used on lumbar curves and some double curves. The TLSO also uses various types of pads to exert pressure on one side of the curve, while the brace itself (often molded a bit higher on one side) will create the counterpressure necessary to keep your body straight.

THE CHARLESTON BRACE

In many parts of the country, a new rigid bracing technique is being tried. Called the Charleston Bending brace, it was developed in 1979 by Dr. Frederick E. Reed, Jr. and C. Ralph Hooper, Jr., C.P.O., both of Charleston, South Carolina. This new brace is similar to a low-profile type, except that it attempts to "overcorrect" the curvature by keeping a patient bent toward the convexity of her curve. According to Dr. Thomas Renshaw, director of Orthopedic Surgery at Newington Children's Hospital in Newington, Connecticut, "Patients can't wear it during the day because they're leaning way over; therefore, it's used only while one sleeps. We first started using it in March of 1986, and since then, we've used it with sixty of our patients who have single and/or flexible curves. At present, its success rate is roughly 80 percent. It looks like a promising technique and further evaluation of its usefulness is going on now." Other studies have been presented to the American Academy of Orthopedic Surgeons, as well as to the Scoliosis Research Society; the success rate indicated in those studies is approximately 83 percent.

WHAT ABOUT ELECTRONIC BRACING?

When I wrote the first edition of *Stopping Scoliosis*, which was published in 1987, electronic bracing, also known as electro-surface stimulation, was still considered by many orthopedists to be a superb alternative to rigid bracing. Early clinical trials showed that the hand-sized devices could stop adolescent curves from progressing roughly 80 percent of the time. What's more, most patients actually *liked* using stimulators: all one had to do was use it every night until one's bones reached maturity, and the little transmit-

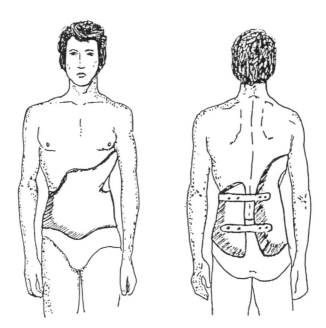

Figure 3.2.   The low-profile brace is usually worn by patients with thoracolumbar and lumbar curves.

ter—which sent mild electric currents through the skin via elec-
trode pads placed on the back over certain muscles—did the rest.
No daytime brace was required.

Unfortunately, in the last few years, this "wonder" device has
fallen out of favor with most orthopedists. Why? "Most of the
recent studies that have been conducted regarding electrical stimulation show it is the same as no treatment at all," says Dr.
Renshaw. "Just why it doesn't work, nobody really knows."

This may come as unsettling news to those who are still being
treated with stimulators. Instead of panicking, however, follow Dr.
Renshaw's sage advice: "If you're being treated with electrical
stimulation and your curve is progressing, you should *stop* treatment and switch to a rigid brace. If you're doing well with electrical stimulation and not ready to stop treatment because of age or
bone maturity, then there's no reason why you can't continue with
it." Another alternative he suggests: "Under an orthopedist's supervision, a patient could stop treatment and see if the curve has
stopped on its own. If it hasn't stopped progressing, the patient
could resume treatment with a rigid brace."

According to Dr. Renshaw, if you're one of those who's being
treated with one of these devices and your curve is not progressing,
there are two possible explanations: first, the curve has stabilized
by itself and probably wouldn't progress anyway; or second, the
treatment may be working. "Many doctors believe that stimulation
may have stopped some people's curves," he says, "but remember,
30 percent of all curves that are treated would stop progressing on
their own, so you can't really prove that treatment with electrical
stimulation stopped the progression."

GETTING USED TO YOUR BRACE

Most youngsters, when faced with having to wear either the Milwaukee or the TLSO brace, have the same question: "How in the
world will I ever get used to wearing this thing?" Many hope that
their doctors will "wean" them into it a few hours at a time until
their bodies and minds can get used to it. Alas, there is no weaning
period. Once your orthotist has adjusted the brace so that it fits
you perfectly, on it goes, for a period of time to be specified by
your doctor. Some patients must wear it daily for about twenty-
three hours, while others can still get good correction by wearing it

twenty hours a day or less. Check with your orthopedist to find out if you're a good candidate for part-time bracing.

Admittedly, the first few days are the worst. You think you'll never be able to tolerate the pelvic girdle squeezing your hips. If you're wearing the underarm type, you'll feel the back of it rub against your shoulder blades, while the bottom portion chafes against your hips and buttocks. If you're wearing a Milwaukee, it will seem as if that pesky neck ring always gets in your way no matter which way you turn. Lean forward, and it pinches your chin; lean back, and those two pads seem to fight you every inch of the way. As for all of those metal bars—well, no matter if you're sitting, standing, or lying down, you feel as if you're being jabbed from every direction. And no matter which type of brace they're wearing, most youngsters can't imagine ever getting used to standing up *that straight!*

You will get used to it, though. As your skin toughens, you'll no longer notice the rubbing and chafing, and any redness will eventually disappear. If you're wearing a Milwaukee brace, you'll find that after a week or so you've trained yourself to avoid the neck ring, but this usually means you'll have to change the way you accomplish certain tasks. For example, if you're currently in school, you'll find that your usual methods for reading and writing—leaning over books or papers—are quite uncomfortable with the Milwaukee brace on. Every time you try to lean forward in your chair, the neck ring will succeed in pulling you back. The best way to solve this problem is to prop up your book so it's nearer eye level, and to move your paper farther away from you on the desk while you're writing. It all takes some getting used to, but it can be done!

In order to feel comfortable with the Milwaukee brace on while you sleep, avoid lying on your stomach—such a position usually results in pressure from the neck ring. Instead, try lying on your side, with a pillow or two propped up behind your back, or on your back, using pillows or other supports beneath your body.

WHAT TO WEAR UNDER THE BRACE

The best way to counteract rubbing and chafing is to wear a T-shirt, leotard, or body stocking beneath your brace. (Girls can continue to wear a bra.) Make sure it fits snugly—excess material causes wrinkles, which will press in on your skin—and that it's seamless. Of course, you can adapt your undergarment to your needs—some kids who wear the underarm brace opt for wearing a tube top that can be pulled down snugly over the hips. If you have a Milwaukee brace, you can trim the arms off the T-shirt, if you like, and snip off excess material around the bottom near the buttocks so that the material doesn't "bunch up" beneath your slacks.

It's a good idea to pick an undergarment that's made of a natural fabric, such as cotton. It will "breathe" and allow excess perspiration to evaporate. Synthetic fabrics, such as nylon or polyester, tend to keep moisture trapped next to the body. Not only will such fabrics make you feel clammy, but the moisture buildup against your skin will soften it and make it more susceptible to sores caused by rubbing.

Many brace wearers prefer to wear undergarments that have been tailor-made for them. Constructed of soft cotton-blend material and considered by many to be more attractive than a standard T-shirt, they're available for males and females. If you wish, you can even order one that has a brassiere built into it. For more information about these unique undergarments—the cost of which is usually covered by medical insurance—write to the Orthotic Undergarment Company, Route 6, Box 46-H, Austin, Texas 78737, and/or Brace Mates, P.O. Box 200, Concord, VA 24538.

One note of caution: never apply body lotions or petroleum jelly to any part of your skin that is covered by the brace, even if you develop slight sores at points on your body where bones— your hipbones, for example—protrude. Lotions and the like are designed to keep the skin moist and soft, and they will make you more susceptible to sores caused by rubbing. If you must, use alcohol to soothe these roughened areas. And if the problem persists, make sure you talk to your doctor about it—it may be that your brace doesn't fit properly.

PROPER FIT

You'll be asked to return to the clinic every three or four months so that your doctor can X ray your spine to see whether or not your curve is progressing, and to see that your brace still fits properly.

Since your body will be growing while you're in the brace, it will be necessary for your doctor to adjust the pressure pads or the pelvic girdle to accommodate this growth. And if you're wearing a Milwaukee brace, he'll have to make adjustments to the bars so that they continue to fit as you grow taller. Some of you will outgrow your brace; in this case, you'll return to the orthotist for a new one.

CLOTHING OVER THE BRACE

For those who are lucky enough to be able to wear the underarm brace, clothing doesn't present much of a problem. Because your neck, shoulders, and chest are free, you can wear the same types of top you've always worn. But since the pelvic girdle will add about an inch to your waist and hips, be prepared to set aside those skin-tight jeans for a while—you'll need slacks that are perhaps one size larger than you're used to. Some youngsters like to wear pants that are elasticized at the waist; they're easier to put on and tend to fit smoothly over the hips. Others who buy fly-front jeans that fit their "new" bodies at the waist and hips often like to have the leg portion taken in so that the pants are properly proportioned all the way down the thighs and legs. You may also want to consider purchasing underpants that are large enough to fit *over* your brace. You'll have an easier time removing them when you go to the bathroom.

If you're wearing a Milwaukee brace, you may be worried about how to cover up the neck ring, and how to conceal the metal bars in front and back. If you're self-conscious, you may want to wear turtleneck tops, or blouses and shirts that are loose-fitting. If wearing such clothing makes you feel better, then go ahead. But bear in mind that a lot of youngsters, sooner or later, don't really care whether they "hide" the hardware or not. They come to accept that they have to wear the brace, and they just wear clothing that makes them feel comfortable. "I wore turtlenecks all year long," said one youngster, "even in hot, muggy weather in the hope that nobody would find out my secret. But guess what? Most of my friends and acquaintances knew I was wearing a brace, and frankly, they didn't care if they saw a little metal encircling my neck. And after sweating it out for several months, I finally decided that my undercover act just wasn't worth the bother. I wore anything I felt like wearing, including V-neck T-shirts and bare-midriff tops! This 'flaunting' of my brace made me feel better about myself—I was proud that I could endure wearing this contraption. I was showing the world that I could handle it. And that's something that not everyone can do!"

WHAT ABOUT ACTIVITIES?

Many youngsters think that because they're going to be wearing a brace many hours a day for several years, all activity will come to a halt. Nothing could be further from the truth! In fact, exercise is extremely important while you're wearing the brace because it helps maintain muscle tone.

You'll probably meet with a physical therapist after you get your brace. She will evaluate your posture, muscles, strength, and flexibility, and talk with you about how active you are right now. Then she'll prescribe specific exercises for you to do every day. Some of these may include push-ups while you're in the brace, or pelvic tilts out of the brace—you lie on the floor and push the small of your back onto it by tightening your abdominal muscles.

WHAT ABOUT SPORTS?

Most doctors encourage brace patients to stay active in sports because they're good for your body and great for your psyche as well.

Although you should check with your doctor about which sports will be best for you, the following are usually considered acceptable, as long as you don't overexert yourself: tennis, Ping-Pong, running, biking, softball, basketball, volleyball, soccer, golf, rowing, and dancing. With your doctor's permission, you probably will be able to swim (without the brace, of course) each day. It is best to avoid contact sports such as football, hockey, and wrestling—these activities could cause you to hurt yourself or someone else, and you could also damage your brace, which would be costly. If you are skilled at sports such as snow skiing or roller skating, your doctor may permit you to continue the activities while in your brace.

WEANING FROM THE BRACE

From the first day you put on the brace, you'll no doubt keep asking your doctor this question: "When can I take it off . . . forever?" His answer will depend on your bone age, how long you've worn the brace, whether you've worn it full-time or part-time, and whether or not your curve has progressed during "confinement."

Let's say that you've been in the brace twenty-three hours a day, every day, for two years, and by looking at your X rays your doctor determines that your curve has either stabilized or progressed only slightly. You're now sixteen years old and, from your doctor's predictions, your bones should stop growing within the next year. To see whether you're ready for "weaning," he'll take an X ray of your spine after you've been out of your brace for about two hours. If within those two hours your spine stays in the same position (which he'll know because he'll take another set of X rays), he'll start weaning you from the brace. For the next three months or so you'll wear it for twenty-one hours. Then the next time you come into the office, he'll take another X ray after you've been out of the brace for four hours. If your spine stays the same after this period, he'll now let you reduce your daily time in the brace to twenty hours. He'll continue this monitoring every three months, increasing your freedom to twelve and then sixteen hours. At the end of a year, if your spine is still straight after being out of the brace for many hours, you'll have to wear it only at night for the last nine months or so. And at the end of that period you'll be free of the brace forever—and chances are good you will have stopped your scoliosis!

WHAT DO KIDS REALLY THINK ABOUT BRACES?

Despite the aggravation that a brace can cause—physically as well as mentally—most youngsters feel that wearing it was worthwhile, and not just because the brace kept their curve from progressing. In many cases, kids feel that the brace makes them feel stronger psychologically. Take Jan Robertson of St. Louis, Missouri, for instance. She wore a Milwaukee brace for nearly two years, but it didn't stop her from being nominated for the Junior Horsewoman of the Year award sponsored by the Missouri Horse Show Association. Says Jan of her experience in the brace, "I think wearing the brace has just made me more determined to succeed at what I do. Wearing it has really taught me a lot about people. I have learned to respect the problems of those who are handicapped and have to spend their lives on crutches or in wheelchairs."

Jan has also learned that people can make wearing the brace difficult, but only if you let them. "Don't let it get you down," she says. "People are always ready to feel sorry for you and to baby you, but they don't really know how to let you be yourself and do the things you have to do. My gym teacher wouldn't let me do anything, but I did anyway. The girls in my gymnastics class were amazed that I could touch my toes with my back completely straight." And how did Jan convince her friends that the brace didn't really make her "different"? She says, "You just have to show them that you're still the same person inside you always were."

A love-hate relationship with her brace

Although she's now twenty-five, Marsha Piepgras has no trouble recalling what it was like wearing her Milwaukee brace from 1977 to 1980, when all youngsters wore braces for twenty-three hours per day. Her story begins in 1976, when she was in sixth grade:

"I didn't know anything about scoliosis then. In fact, on the day that the school nurse screened us, I didn't have any idea why I was being asked to bend over. She checked out my back and then called in another nurse. They mumbled something about my having a slight curvature, but said it was probably nothing to worry about. I took their word for it.

"By the time I was in seventh grade I knew a little bit about scoliosis. One of the girls in my class was wearing a back brace, and we all knew it was because she had a curvature in her spine. So when it came time to be screened that year, I had some idea of what they were looking for when they asked me to bend over. Of course, I was afraid that if they found a curvature, I'd have to wear a brace just like hers.

"When the exam was over, the nurse told me she thought I had scoliosis, and that she'd be sending a letter home to my mother. I came home bawling that day—I thought for sure I had it. I felt terrible!

"But when we got the letter, all it said was that in scoliosis screening they noticed I had something called a 'thoracic hump.' That was all the letter said. I thought to myself, 'Oh, this is something different. This isn't scoliosis.' I tried to talk myself out of it, I guess, and I told kids at school that it wasn't scoliosis after all. But when we went to my family doctor, he took an X ray. Sure enough, I had scoliosis. I was devastated. All I could think about was I'd have to wear a brace. So my mom and I made an appointment with a specialist to find out what would have to happen next.

"I was pretty nervous when I met the specialist, but he tried to reassure me by saying that just because I had scoliosis, it didn't mean I'd have to wear a brace. He said he'd take an X ray of my spine to see how it looked. Then all of us together would decide what to do.

"When the X ray came back from the lab, the doctor put it up to the light and I could see the curve for myself. I was really upset, because I felt fine, yet I could see how my spine had curved into an S shape. I couldn't feel it, but there it was, crooked! He explained that because both parts of the curve measured 26 degrees—the top and bottom—it was a 'balanced' curve. He said it wasn't that bad, and that we wouldn't have to do anything for now. We could come back in three months and he'd check it again to see if it had gotten worse. I was so relieved! Maybe I wouldn't have to wear a brace after all!

"When we went back to his office three months later, I had more X rays taken. My curve had gotten bigger—the top was now 36 degrees, and the bottom was 18 degrees. Now my curve was unbalanced. And because it had increased in just three months, it would probably keep getting worse—unless I was put into a Milwaukee brace.

"As soon as he said that, I wanted to bawl my head off. I was really scared! I didn't want to have any part of it at all. I figured that if I had to wear it, nobody would like me. As a seventh grader, I was just starting to realize that boys were pretty interesting, and I figured if I had to wear a brace, I'd never have a boyfriend. That seems silly to me now, but then it was really important.

"I kept thinking about that girl who wore a brace at school. Everybody thought she was weird—mostly because she had a terrible personality—but I really thought people would think of me like her. I didn't get much time to dwell on that, because before I knew it, I was in the cast room being fitted for the brace.

"It was awful! The room seemed like it was 95 degrees, and I hated standing there while they put on the plaster. All I could think about was getting this over with and going home. Then I wouldn't have to think about it until the brace was ready—in about two weeks.

"They had a lot of trouble fitting the brace to me. I spent an entire day going between the doctor and the brace people, what with all the adjustments they had to make. Then they gave me the wrong brace—it belonged to another girl, but nobody knew it for several hours. They kept trying to adjust it to fit me, but of course it wouldn't. Finally somebody figured out that they had the wrong brace, and they finally located the one that was intended for me. By the time they all finished working me over, I was really uncomfortable, but at least it fit!

"I felt so awkward trying to get into the car to go home. I couldn't just hop in the way I used to. Now I had to sort of slide into the seat, and when I finally got in, I felt like I couldn't breathe—that neck ring really pinched me under the chin! All the way home I stared at the ceiling of the car and wondered how I'd ever get used to wearing this thing. How would I ever face the kids at school?

"When I woke up the next morning, I took one look at the brace and decided no way, I just could not face the idea of having to go to school with it. It was almost the end of the school year, and I thought if I could just avoid wearing it for another month or so, nobody would ever have to know.

"Mom and I fought constantly. At first she tried being sympathetic about it. She'd say, 'I know you don't like this. I understand, but you've just got to wear it.' I refused to listen to her. I simply wasn't going to wear it.

"Finally, just to keep the peace, I agreed to wear it—but only when I slept. Mom got so frustrated with me that she called the clinic and got the names of twin girls who'd had scoliosis and worn braces, and she made me go over to their house to talk. I think she thought this would make me feel better—seeing other girls who had the same problem—but actually it didn't help me much. As it turned out, the girls had just gotten out of their braces. There they sat, with perfectly straight backs and no braces. That would never be me, I thought. And besides, they were seventeen. I was twelve. I had such a long time to go in the brace!

"After that, my mom tried again to help. This time she found a young woman in her twenties who'd had surgery for scoliosis and arranged for us to have dinner together. Maybe she thought it would scare me into wearing the brace.

"That was the first time I'd worn the brace out in public. Talking to that woman didn't really help me, but getting out did. I kept thinking everybody in the restaurant was staring at me, but after a while it didn't bother me as much. That was the best thing I could have done—making the first move to wear it outside and seeing people's reaction to it. That summer I occasionally wore the brace in public, but I still wore it mostly when I slept.

"When I started eighth grade that fall, I had resolved that I was going to have to wear it because it wasn't going to go away. That first day of eighth grade was the hardest of my life, because I knew if I didn't wear it that day, I never would.

"I got through the first day all right, and then everything was okay. I wore turtlenecks to try and hide it as much as possible, but the kids at school could still see it underneath my clothes. They weren't negative about it at all—just inquisitive. Everybody wanted to know what it was for, and how I could sleep with it on. As time went on, more and more people knew about it, and I eventually quit trying to hide it with clothes. I became bolder and just didn't care about it that much.

"I wore the brace pretty regularly during eighth and ninth grade, and finally, when I started tenth grade, the doctor said I could be weaned from it. My curves were now at 25 and 18 degrees, and they stabilized even when I was out of the brace for hours at a time. For several months I only had to wear it for sixteen hours a day. Eventually I only had to wear it at night.

"At last the day came when my orthopedist said I didn't have to wear it anymore. You'd think I would have been ecstatic about it, but I wasn't! I'd gotten so used to sleeping with it on that I couldn't bear to be without it! Would you believe I still continued wearing it at night for three more whole months? I'd really gotten to like the support the brace gave me. In fact, I felt like I was melting into the bed without it. I actually couldn't fall asleep without it!

"When I told my doctor about it, he put his foot down and said I couldn't be so dependent on the brace, that eventually I'd get used to sleeping without it. Of course he was right, but I sure had a hard time going along with it. To this day—I go back to the clinic every year to have an X ray—he still calls me his 'star patient,' his 'champion brace wearer.' And when he introduces me to doctors visiting at the clinic, he always likes to refer to me as 'the girl who liked her brace so much she didn't want to take it off.'

"It seems funny now, especially since I had so much trouble getting used to the brace in the beginning. But I think the whole experience taught me a lot about myself. Wearing a brace made me go through something at a young age—it was something I *had* to accept. A lot of kids aren't faced with something hard like that. But I was forced to deal with it and had to learn to look at the good side of things. I couldn't just sit there and feel sorry for myself. I finally had to realize that it was still me inside the brace, that it didn't really matter. It helped to talk to people about it, to explain things to them. Once you bring it out in the open, it makes it easier for you and for them."

Tears first, then acceptance

Diane Borgen has had more than her share of medical problems. When she was only a year and a half old, she had surgery to repair a hip that was dislocated at birth, and she later developed kidney infections that would plague her for several of her childhood years. When she was screened for scoliosis in sixth grade, at age twelve, the school nurse noticed that one of her shoulders seemed higher than the other. "It looked like I had a lump on my back," recalls Diane, "and I immediately thought it was cancer. I'd had so many problems with my body up to that point, it wouldn't have surprised me if it had been cancer. Even so, I was really scared!"

Diane and her parents made an appointment with the family doctor who assured them that Diane's problem wasn't cancer. It was scoliosis. He referred them to a scoliosis specialist in another city. Diane had X rays taken; then came the verdict: she had a 21-degree curvature. "It was just another blow," says Diane's mother, Pat. "Diane had had so many medical problems, all of them major. But each problem had been corrected, and we just hoped that this one would follow the same path."

When the orthopedist told the Borgens that Diane would have to wear a Milwaukee brace for several years to keep the curve from progressing, Diane burst into tears. "It was really difficult for me to accept. Since I'd had this history of problems, it seemed like everything about me was bad. This was just one more problem, and I kept wondering, 'Why me?' I kept right on crying as my parents tried to comfort me. They kept trying to make me feel better by reminding me that some kids can't walk, some kids have braces on their teeth. And they tried to encourage me by saying that if the doctor could help me in some way, I should take him up on it. I knew they were right, but I didn't like hearing about it. Why did I have to go through this?"

"Eventually I started to calm down—I guess I resigned myself to the fact that I could handle this problem, too. But then my doctor showed me a picture of the brace. I took one look at it and started crying again. I thought it would hurt me . . . or choke me. It was just soooo straight!

"Being fitted for the brace, having the plaster mold put on, was terrible at first. I didn't like wearing that slinky body stocking. It was so revealing! And it was uncomfortable holding on to the bar while they put on the plaster. My arms really ached. The best part was when they cut the mold apart with a little saw—it was fun seeing the shape of my body in the plaster.

"When we picked up the brace from the shop a few weeks later, I put it on immediately. It felt really weird, almost like a machine. And I had a lot of trouble putting it on by myself. It probably took a month before I could do it without somebody helping me.

"I was pretty embarrassed wearing the brace during the first week of school, but my friends and teachers pretty much accepted it. I wore turtlenecks for a while, but since everybody in school knew about the brace anyway, I eventually quit trying to hide it. Another girl in my class wore one, but she'd always try to cover hers and pretend it wasn't there. She wouldn't talk to people about it. I could see she was making things uncomfortable for herself and other people, and I didn't want that to happen to me. So I was pretty open about it, and that helped a lot.

"I kept active while I was wearing the brace. I'd play softball with it on and even wore it on a trip to Hawaii. In fact, I got to the point where I felt best with it on—I'd feel like a noodle when I took it off.

"Every three months I had to go back to the clinic for X rays. Each time the curve had gotten progressively worse. When it reached 40 degrees—what all the doctors call the 'magic number'— I started to worry that I might have to have surgery. That was a big fear, so I did my brace exercises a ton of times, hoping they'd help. I think they did, because my curve has stayed right around 40 degrees to this day.

"My parents really helped me through it. They always went with me to the doctor and would encourage me to do my exercises and to wear the brace twenty-three hours a day. They kept telling me the doctor knew what he was doing, and that the brace would help me. If they would have questioned it, I would have, too. But they accepted it, and so did I.

"A lot of my parents' friends would say to them, 'How can you make your daughter wear it? It's ruining her life.' But Mom and Dad would say, 'You don't know Diane. She's got a great attitude and she can handle it.' It made me feel good to know they had a lot of confidence in me. I might have had some real serious psychological problems if it hadn't been for them."

No big deal at all

Nineteen-year-old Elise Nelson is the kind of youngster who doesn't let anything—including scoliosis—get her down. In fact, when she met her orthopedist and he told her that she had an S-curve, 20 degrees at the top and bottom, she wasn't worried a bit. "The news that I had scoliosis didn't have much of an effect on me," she says. "My curve wasn't very big at first, and my doctor said he'd watch it over the next three months. He said if it increased, I could probably use a stimulator. That sounded okay to me. Actually, I thought it might be kind of fun."

When Elise returned for X rays three months later, her curve had indeed increased: the top now measured 29 degrees; the bottom,

21. "The doctor showed me a little model of a Milwaukee brace," she says. "The thought of wearing it didn't bother me at all. It was no big deal.

"Of course, I was pretty nervous when they put the plaster mold on me—two college-aged orthopedic residents were doing it, and I was only wearing a body stocking. So it was pretty embarrassing, but they told jokes and kidded me a lot, which made it a lot easier.

"It didn't bother me to have to wear the brace to school. In fact, I was actually glad that I had to wear a neck ring. I figured that if people could see part of the brace, they'd know what was going on. I liked the fact that it was so obvious. I think it helped people understand what I was going through.

"Nobody ever made fun of me that I can remember, but the first day I wore it, kids at school seemed scared to say anything to me. Eventually word got around behind my back that I was wearing a brace because I had scoliosis, and then I was treated just like everybody else.

"I have to admit it: sometimes it made me feel self-conscious. But it also gave me an excuse. Sometimes teenagers feel like they have to do everything that everybody else is doing; they feel like they have to be part of the crowd. When I didn't want to be part of the crowd, or if I wasn't feeling too popular anyway, I could always blame the brace. I know it was unrealistic to think that way, but somehow it helped me feel better about myself when I was feeling insecure or unpopular.

"I didn't give up any activities because of the brace. I took dancing—ballet, tap, and jazz. I got permission from my orthopedist to take off the brace for an hour during the day so I could practice dancing. He said the exercise would help strengthen my back. I even started cheerleading while I was in it. I didn't do anything incredibly daring, mind you, but I could do most of the cheers and some of the jumps. Of course, sometimes the brace got in my way—like the first time I tried to play softball in it. The coach put me out in center field and the batter hit a grounder to me. I squatted down and fell face first in the dirt! It was the most embarrassing moment of my life! But I'd probably have felt that way even if I hadn't been wearing a brace at the time.

"In the three years and two months that I wore the brace, the only thing that bugged me was how my parents and grandparents would sometimes treat me. They'd give me special treatment. If I bent over to pick something up, they say, 'Oh, don't do that, you'll hurt your back.' I guess they thought I wasn't capable of doing normal things. But I just felt like I could do anything! And I pretty much did everything I wanted to. I just had to show them that I wasn't an invalid.

"Today my curves are 21 and 17, and I don't have to wear the brace anymore. I feel good and look good. The brace made me feel better about myself, because it's not something everybody can get through."

4

Surgical Treatments
For Adolescents and Adults with Curves of 40 Degrees and Beyond

This chapter examines many of the surgical techniques that are available today, providing you with a fairly graphic picture of what orthopedic surgeons actually do in the operating room in the process of straightening out a curve. In Chapter 6 you'll meet youngsters and adults who've had operations to correct their scoliosis, all of whom will tell you about their surgical experience in their own words. In most cases, they have been extremely candid about their emotions, frustrations, and their pain, both psychological and physical.

Before you delve into this chapter, however, you need to know that your state of mind can have an important effect on the amount of distress you experience before and after surgery, and that it can even affect your rate of recovery. For some people, knowing "all there is to know" about surgery improves their state of mind. It makes them feel that they're in control of the situation. For others, the motto "Ignorance is bliss" holds true. The less they know about the surgery, the better they can cope with it. If you belong in the second category, skip to Chapter 5.

RELAXATION TECHNIQUES

The first thing to know is this: even under the best of circumstances, the prospect of surgery is going to cause anxiety, so it's an
especially good time to consider making use of a relaxation technique, such as meditation or muscle relaxation. Researchers have
found that relaxation can be beneficial in lowering heart rate and
blood pressure, boosting the immune system, and decreasing the
amount of distress you feel.

If you find yourself fretting about surgery in the days or weeks
before it, you may want to try the following technique to limit
worry that was developed by Dr. Thomas D. Borkovec and his
colleagues at the Pennsylvania State University:

- Learn to identify worrisome thoughts that are unnecessary or
  unpleasant.

- Establish a half hour of "worry time" to take place at the same
  time and same place each day.

- If you find yourself worrying at various other times of the day,
  try to postpone the worry to that half hour you've scheduled as
  "worry time" and then try to get absorbed in other activities.

DIFFERENT SURGICAL TECHNIQUES

If you ask an orthopedic surgeon to describe the surgical technique
for correcting scoliosis, it's likely that he'll interrupt you and ask,
"Which one?" Today there are dozens of different ways to correct
scoliosis, and each technique has its own special benefits and risks.
Before we explore the five most common procedures used across
the country, let's step back into time to 1911 when Russell Hibbs,
an orthopedic surgeon at the New York Orthopaedic Hospital in
New York City, performed the world's first spinal fusion. We'll let
Dr. Hugo A. Keim, a spine surgeon at this hospital, now a part of
the Columbia-Presbyterian Medical Center, tell us how spine surgery got its start:

> In 1911, it was unbelievable that anyone even considered
> doing spine surgery. Doctors then just used 'drop' ether, and

that didn't always keep the patient asleep. They had no blood replacement products and no antibiotics to guard against infection. In fact, when Russell Hibbs proposed the idea of doing a spine fusion on a person who had tuberculosis, everybody thought he was a maniac! He couldn't become a member of the American Orthopedic Association—the members blackballed him because they thought he was crazy!

Hibbs didn't use rods and wire fixations—he just fused the spine. But because he had no way to keep the spine straight while it healed—the job that rods and wires do today—he took two or three vertebrae at a time, welding them together by using little chips of bone taken from the spine. This meant that he had to bring a patient into surgery, do two or three fusions, close up the incisions, put her in a plaster cast, and keep her in the hospital six to eight weeks while she healed. Then he'd have to go back in and do another two or three vertebrae, finish the job, put on another cast, leave her on her back for another six to eight weeks, and repeat this routine until all of the curved vertebrae were fused. Believe it or not, the average patient in those days was here in the hospital for a whole year!

Russell Hibbs paved the way for the kinds of spine operations we do today. Although he was initially considered a complete whacko by his peers, his pioneering work as a surgeon would eventually be hailed as brilliant, and the medical community realized that much could be learned from him."

Surgeons today owe a great debt to Dr. Hibbs, but as you'll see, they've added some highly sophisticated techniques to spinal fusions. As a result, spine surgery today is far more complex—but more successful—than at any other time in history.

The Harrington Rod Technique

Developed in Texas in the 1940s by the late Dr. Paul Harrington of Houston, the *Harrington rod technique* is still used on people who have idiopathic scoliosis. Though he was not the first to propose the use of metal "fixation," he invented spinal hardware that has stood the test of time and is the standard by which other types are judged.

Some surgeons consider this the easiest—and the safest—of all techniques because it is done posteriorly—that is, from the back. (Other techniques are performed anteriorly—from the front or side of the body—and will be discussed later.) If your curve is 40 degrees or more, a Harrington rod may be all or a part of your surgeon's intrumentation of choice. (See Figure 4.1.)

Once the surgeon has made his midline incision, he and his assistants will inject a solution that is designed to slow down bleeding into your back muscles. Then they separate the muscles, holding them back with special metal clamps so that your spine is in clear view.

The sequence of events that follows will vary from surgeon to surgeon, and the number of steps will vary depending upon whether you have a single or a double curve. Instead of recording all the possible variations, we'll examine just one commonly used step by step approach for a single C curve; it will give you a basic understanding of what's being done and why.

Once the spine is exposed, the surgeon will begin the process of straightening, or "distracting," your curve. Between the two vertebrae located at the highest and lowest points of a curve, he'll insert a *hook*—an L-shaped piece of metal that has an opening on one end. Into these openings, he'll insert an *outrigger*, a rod-shaped device that operates much like a car jack; as the surgeon "cranks" the outrigger, the rod extends and straightens the spine in the process.

While the outrigger holds your spine in place, the surgeon will begin to "prepare" your spine for the bone graft that will fuse to it. He will remove the outer bone, or *cortex*, of each vertebra involved in the curve. By decorticating the vertebrae, the surgeon can expose the living bone that's underneath, a spongy, porous sort of bone that releases blood, the life-giving ingredient that will help your spine—and the bone graft that's going to be inserted—fuse together into a solid mass of bone.

Once your vertebrae have been decorticated, the spine is ready for the insertion of the Harrington rod. The surgeon will remove the outrigger and insert the new rod into the hooks. It also contains ratchets, which can be "jacked up" to straighten your spine to the point where your surgeon is satisfied with the correction. In most cases, a Harrington rod can be extended to a point where

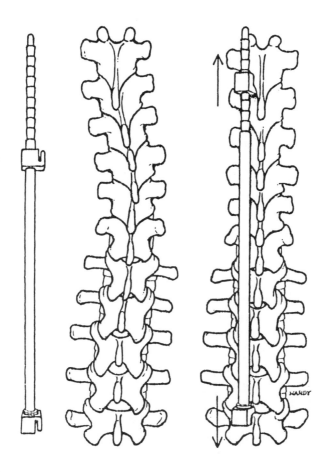

Figure 4.1. The Harrington rod implant is considered by some surgeons to be the easiest and safest of all surgical techniques for idiopathic scoliosis. This Harrington distraction rod lengthens the curve.

your curve will be straightened by about 60 percent; in other words, if you entered the operating room with a curve of 60 degrees, by the time the surgeon finishes extending the Harrington rod, your curve will have been reduced to about 24 degrees.

Why can't surgeons, using the Harrington technique, reduce curves to zero? The answer lies just beneath the bumpy spinous processes of your vertebral column: situated there is the delicate *spinal cord,* a thick ropelike structure made of nerve tissue that is the sensitive pathway by which your brain sends messages to various parts of your body.

As your surgeon distracts your spine, he is manipulating your spinal cord as well, a very risky maneuver. "The spinal cord is very unforgiving of any bumping, however slight," warns Dr. Lonstein. "When it is bumped, you can either become paraplegic [paralysis of the lower body, including both legs] or become partially paralyzed, losing the function of one leg. And if the spinal cord is stretched too much during distraction, you can interfere with the blood circulation in the cord, and this can also cause paralysis. This is why, with any method of distraction, the correction is considered maximum at 60 percent."

Knowing now just how risky distraction can be, you might ask, "How does the surgeon know how much pressure to use when straightening my spine?" Unfortunately, there are no easy answers to this question, no scientific tables listing pounds of pressure that a surgeon should exert on a person's spine. (At least one scientist tried to develop guidelines, but they proved to be ineffective.) Indeed, Dr. Keim willingly admits that safe distraction of the spine is not a science, but rather a delicate art: "It's like asking how much pressure you should put on your toothbrush when you're brushing your teeth. Or how hard you should wipe your eye when you get sand in it. If you rub too hard, you can damage your eye; if you don't rub hard enough, you can't get rid of the sand. Distraction is a delicate thing, something you learn after you do hundreds and hundreds of surgeries. It's part of the art of medicine, and surgeons get a 'feel' for what's right and how far to straighten the spine, but it takes years and years of experience."

Next, using a special tool, your surgeon will begin collecting bone graft material from either your hip or your ribs. He'll move aside, or "reflect," the muscles that surround either of these structures, then remove small strips of bone with a special tool. The bone is then cut into hundreds of match-sized strips, which are packed in a criss-cross fashion from the top to the bottom of the decorticated vertebrae. After four to six months in adolescents and six to twelve months or longer in adults, these tiny chips will meld together into one solid piece of bone. Says Dr. Keim of the eventual fusion: "It's beautiful. It looks like someone poured molten wax over the spine. You cannot distinguish between the individual strips of bone. What you really end up with is a single, smooth, elongated section of vertebrae."

When all the chips of bone have been laid in, the surgical team will be ready to finish the job they started perhaps two or three hours earlier. They'll remove the clamps that held back your muscles during surgery, and smooth the muscles and other tissues back over your newly straightened spine. Finally, they close up the incision with sutures, and you're off to the recovery room. Patients who receive Harrington rods can expect to wear a postsurgical brace for four to six months.

Variations on the Harrington Rod

Depending upon the type of curve you have, your surgeon may elect to do more than insert a single Harrington rod. For example, if you have a particularly stubborn curve, he may insert two rods: a Harrington on the concave side to distract it, and a "compression" rod on the convex side, which actually pulls the bowed sides of the vertebrae together. When used together, these rods straighten your spine from two directions, and can often provide better correction than if only one rod is used.

In cases where a patient's bones are particularly soft, it's possible that the hooks of a Harrington rod could break through the vertebrae to which they're attached. To ensure that this doesn't happen, a surgeon will often hold the rod in place with wires. This wiring technique can be done in many different ways, and your surgeon probably will have developed his own method. Some surgeons thread their wires through the neural canal and then twist them around the Harrington; others, such as Dr. Keim, prefer to drill small holes through the spinous processes, place the wire through the holes, and then tighten them around the rod(s). This latter technique and variations of it are considered safest, since the wires do not pass through the canal that surrounds the spinal cord.

The Luque-Type Procedure

To alleviate some of the potential problems associated with the Harrington rod—hooks breaking through weak vertebrae and spinal cords being stretched beyond their natural limits—various techniques have been developed. Many orthopedic surgeons today are using an implant procedure developed in the early 1970s by surgeon Eduardo Luque of Mexico City. The *Luque* (pronounced "loo-key") *technique* does not use hooks or Harrington-type rods; instead, many wires are threaded through the neural canal and then twisted around two thin rods placed on either side of the curved vertebrae. Since there are a number of variations on the Luque technique, all with different names, we'll simply refer to this wiring method as a Luque-type procedure. (See Figure 4.2.)

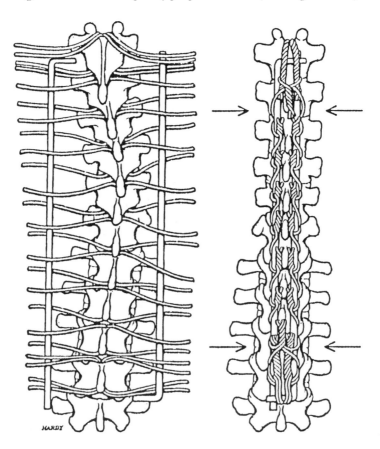

Figure 4.2. A Luque-type implant consists of two L-shaped rods, plus many wires that are passed through the neural or spinal canal. When wiring is complete, the ends are twisted and turned down.

Your surgeon will expose your spine in the same fashion as he would for a Harrington rod insert—he makes his incision in the middle of your back, injects your muscles with solution, gently separates them, and holds them back with clamps. He will also remove the outer bone or cortex of the vertebrae involved in the curve because later on he will need a "live" surface to which he will apply bone graft.

Once he finishes decorticating your vertebrae, he will remove what's called the *ligamentum flavum*—the rubbery fibers that connect one vertebra to another—so that he has an opening through which he can eventually pass the wires through the neural canal.

Now your surgeon will thread all the wires through the neural canal and pull them around the bony ring of each vertebra involved in the curvature. Then he'll take the first *L-rod* (so-called because of its shape) and bend it slightly so that it will conform to the natural contours of your spine. That done, he'll place the rod, which acts as a lever, between the spinous and transverse processes, and push it toward the center while twisting the wires around it to hold it in place. He will repeat this procedure using a second L-rod on the opposite side. After all the wires have been twisted and your spine has been straightened, the surgical team will turn down the ends of the twisted wires to keep them from protruding.

Small chips of bone will be removed from your hip or ribs and your surgeon will place them lengthwise along the outer edges of the rods. This bone graft will eventually fuse to the vertebrae and strengthen them. Since the two rods and the network of wiring provide considerable strength, there is usually no need to wear a brace after surgery.

Although surgeons who use a Luque-type procedure believe they get a stronger fixation than they could with Harrington—and of course their patients are delighted that they don't have to wear braces—there is a considerable amount of risk involved. As we've discussed, damaging the spinal cord is a hazard in any scoliosis surgery, but Luque-type procedures pose a special danger, because wires are passed through the neural canal, which contains the spinal cord.

In fact, there are surgeons who are highly critical of the "wire fixation" trend. While critics admit that a Luque-type procedure is particularly beneficial for people who have neurological deficits or defects that result in soft spinal bone, they usually voice two complaints. First, because the wires come in contact with the spinal cord, there is high neurological risk. Second, because of all the metal and wires used, there is less area available for bone graft, and thus less area that will solidify.

According to Drs. Ben Allen, Jr. and Ron Ferguson, scoliosis specialists at the Shriners' Hospital for Crippled Children in Greenville, South Carolina, who developed a Luque procedure of their own called the *Galveston technique,* their procedure has never caused permanent paralysis. The two surgeons themselves have used it on hundreds of people, and they've also documented the results of more than 500 operations performed by orthopedists using the technique at Stanford University, Indiana University, Northwestern University, the Cleveland Clinic, and Newington Children's Hospital in Connecticut. "In these cases," says Dr. Allen, "only two patients experienced slight spinal cord problems—nothing more than a tingling in the legs—and there were no long-term complications. Thus far, our method appears to be as safe as the Harrington implant or other methods currently in use."

The Cotrel-Dubousset Technique

Surgeons, always trying to develop new and better ways of straightening spines, often wind up selecting certain elements of proven techniques, such as the Harrington or the Luque, and adding new twists of their own. One of the newest and most popular developments is called the *Cotrel-Dubousset* or *C-D technique,* named for the French surgeons Yves Cotrel and Jean Dubousset, who developed it. Used for the first time in the United States in September 1984, this method is said to employ the best part of the Harrington—its safety factor—with the best of the Luque—the strength from two rods and an increased number of attachment points. The C-D is considered to be an extremely *stable* implant technique that not only corrects a curve from the front and side, but also derotates it.

If your surgeon uses this technique, he'll expose and prepare your spine as if he were going to perform a Harrington or a Luque. But instead of using just two hooks at the top and bottom of the curve, he'll insert several hooks along your spine and attach one

Luque-type rod to the concave side. Once this rod is in place, the surgeon can use a special tool that derotates or uncurls the spine as it straightens it; he'll use tiny screws to lock the rod into the hooks so that the corrected spine stays in position. He'll then attach a second rod to the convex side of the curve to compress it. These two rods are held together by smaller connection rods that cross them and form a rectangular shape. Finally, your surgeon will apply tiny bone chips along the spine so that it fuses solidly. In most cases, because the spine has been fortified with so much hardware, there is no need to wear a brace after surgery.

A Word About "No-Brace" Techniques

As you can imagine, Luque-type and Cotrel-Dubousset procedures are extremely popular with patients because there's usually no need to wear a brace after surgery. In fact, I wouldn't be a bit surprised if surgical candidates reading this book were already planning to march into the hospital and plead with their surgeons to perform one or the other of these. Before you do that, please take a moment and contemplate these wise statements made by some of America's most highly respected orthopedic surgeons.

Says Dr. James Ogilvie of the Twin Cities Scoliosis Spine Center:

> With a Luque or a Galveston, you're entering the spinal canal, so in order to perform the procedure correctly and safely, it takes a much different skill level on the part of the surgeon. Just as the Luque or the Galveston is not for every patient, so are these techniques not for every surgeon.

Dr. Robert Winter of the Minnesota Spine Center also offers a warning:

> Let's say a young girl with idiopathic scoliosis comes into the clinic and, based on my assessment of her condition, I tell her that my number one choice is to do a Harrington and put her in a brace for six months. And let's say she says, "I don't want the brace. I've heard about a new operation. Can you do that instead?" My answer will be, "Yes, I can do that, but Harrington is still my first choice." "Why?" she'll ask. "Well, I have to pass all those wires in there, and that increases the

risk rate considerably." Most patients will say, "I don't want to take that risk. I'll have the Harrington and wear the brace."

But if a patient persists and says, "I don't care. I can't stand the thought of that brace. I'll take the risk," then I'd probably do the surgery—but first, she's going to have to sign an informed consent form that says I've informed her of the risk and that she's accepted it.

There are occasions where I firmly believe that if she wants a certain type of instrumentation and I don't think that is the right one for her curvature, I'll say, "It's not the right thing to do." Take an adult patient whose bone is quite soft—I don't care if you put in a Harrington, Luque, or Cotrel, it has a higher tendency to pop out of place if the bone is soft and therefore the wearing of a brace is ultraimportant to that kind of patient. But if this patient still insisted that I do it, I'd tell her she'd have to find another doctor. And her chances of finding someone who would do the surgery are pretty good.

If you're contemplating spine surgery, I urge you to think about what these experts have said before you get too "hung up" on one technique or another. From all the research I've done, I've come to the conclusion, as have many surgeons across the country, that there isn't one single technique that will work on everyone, nor is there one procedure that is "the best." I've also discovered that there are surgeons out there who will tout just one technique as being superior to all others. Moreover, if you didn't hear the experts' message loud and clear: *all surgeons do not enter the operating room with the same level of skill.*

For all these reasons, make sure you are aware of all of the risks involved in the surgery that will be performed on you and your particular condition, that you find out why a particular procedure is being recommended, that you seek a second opinion if you are in doubt, and that you select a surgeon who has a great deal of experience with scoliosis surgery. Says one orthopedic surgeon who wished to remain anonymous: "It's a delicate subject to talk about, but the results from some of these surgical techniques are absolutely bizarre. One scoliosis center will report 15 percent trouble with one procedure, and another center will report absolutely no trouble whatsoever. That, I think, is a technique problem. Some surgeons are not as skilled as other surgeons. And if you look at a surgeon who's had problems with his surgical patients, it'll be someone who's only done fifteen cases. Of course, as he or she gets better at it, the problems disappear. But the point is, a surgical patient needs to be in expert, practiced hands. You don't want to be a guinea pig."

This is intelligent advice for anyone thinking about surgery, and it applies to the following surgical technique as well.

The Dwyer Technique

In the 1960s, Australian orthopedic surgeon Alan Dwyer developed a very dramatic surgical technique, performed near the front of the body, that is sometimes used on people who have severe or inflexible curves. In this procedure, instead of distracting the spine and fusing all the vertebrae involved in the curve, the surgeon removes several discs located between vertebrae at the top or apex of a curve, inserts bone graft into the remaining spaces, and compresses the outer edges of these vertebrae with a special cable system that derotates and straightens the spine.

Because this is an anterior (front) technique, a patient will be positioned on his side so that the surgeon can easily make the incision that may, depending upon the location of the curve, begin just beneath the shoulder blade, slope across the side of the rib cage, and end near the groin. Once the incision is complete, the surgical team will inject into surrounding tissues a solution that slows bleeding. Then they'll separate muscles from fat layers and hold them back with clamps so that they can approach the spine.

In order to get a clear view of the spine, the surgeon and his assistants will remove a rib and a certain amount of cartilage, and then move aside such organs as the liver, kidney, spleen, and lung. Once the spine is exposed, the team will begin removing the rubbery discs that are wedged between the vertebrae at the top of the curve. For reasons that are not completely understood, these discs hold a curve in a locked position, and by removing them, the curve can be more easily manipulated.

Now the surgeon is ready to insert the *Dwyer instrumentation*.

Onto the side of each vertebra involved, he'll fasten a thin metal cap that has a hole in the center of it. Next he'll insert a screw through the hole and rotate it until it reaches the opposite side of the vertebra. He'll repeat these steps with all the necessary vertebrae.

At this point, a strong but flexible metal cable will be drawn through openings in the tops of the screws, and chips of bone (taken from the rib that was removed earlier) will be inserted into the spaces once occupied by the discs. These bone chips will eventually fuse to the inner walls of the vertebrae to form a solid bone mass.

Using a tool called a *cable tensioner,* the surgeon will now tighten the cable and as he does so, your vertebrae will be pulled together, thus straightening your spine. To make sure that the cable remains secure, the surgeon will crimp the screw heads at each end of the cable. Finally, he will return all your organs to their original positions and close the incision.

Depending upon the severity of a curve, a surgeon might elect to perform the *Dwyer technique* to derotate it first, then perform a second posterior surgery to straighten the curve. In these cases, the second surgery may be performed on the same day, or may occur a week or two later. In some cases, patients who've been corrected by the Dwyer technique must wear a brace for four to six months after surgery.

The Zielke Technique

Like other surgeons who have tried to improve upon the instrumentation designed by their predecessors or peers, Klaus Zielke of Germany developed a surgical technique that is fast becoming the *preferred* anterior technique. It mimics the Dwyer, but has a special feature all its own—Zielke's system uses a flexible rod instead of a cable and employs a specially designed tool that helps the surgeon derotate the spine with relative ease while it simultaneously straightens the curve. In many cases, patients who have had a Zielke will not have to undergo a second surgery to complete the correction of their curves, but they may have to wear a brace until their spines heal.

All the preliminary steps leading up to exposure of the spine are identical to those involved with Dwyer. Once your spine is in clear view, the surgeons will also remove the appropriate discs and ligaments before they begin to install the instrumentation.

As you can see in Figure 4.3, the *Zielke technique* does not require that the surgeon cap the sides of your vertebrae with metal plates. Instead, he begins by preparing a small opening on the side of each involved vertebra, into which he will insert a screw with a U-shaped head or nut. Just like the Dwyer, the Zielke screws are rotated through the center of each vertebra. At the first and last vertebra involved, the surgeon will position another type of screw that will be used for securing the ends of the rod after the curve has been derotated and straightened.

Next a flexible rod is threaded through the tops of the screws and the derotation bar is put into position. By pulling the lever handle, the surgeon can now derotate and straighten the spine. Then he will take bone chips from the rib and wedge them into the

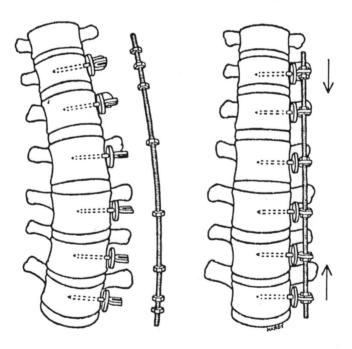

Figure 4.3. When a Zielke implant is used, a flexible rod is threaded through the tops of screws inserted into the vertebrae. A special attachment (not shown) derotates and straightens the spine.

disc spaces. That done, he will tighten the nuts on the screws, remove the derotating bar, and close the incision.

Surgeons' Comments About Dwyer/Zielke

If you think these two anterior approaches seem formidable and complicated, you're absolutely right. They are, and no competent surgeon in the world would try to tell you otherwise. But at present, orthopedists who specialize in scoliosis surgery seem to be divided in their points of view concerning the effectiveness of and, more important, the risk involved with the Dwyer and Zielke techniques. Consider the strong viewpoint of Dr. Winter, a world-renowned scoliosis surgeon who has performed hundreds of anterior surgeries:

> The Dwyer and Zielke operations have changed the whole ball game of scoliosis surgery. Designed to treat curves of 40 to 70 degrees, they reduce the number of bones that have to be operated on. In fact, it's quite possible in some curves to take out just two discs, work on three vertebrae, and completely wipe out the curve. With each disc, you can fix a deformity by about 15 degrees, so by taking three discs out, you can change a 45-degree curve to zero. The correction we get is infinitely better than we could ever get before.
>
> Despite the fairly long incision, and pushing the kidney and other organs out of the way, patients do very well. It's a very low blood loss operation and patients seem to have less pain with Dwyer and Zielke than they do with Harrington or Cotrel-Dubousset.
>
> I think the risk rate is very low, and there's less chance of paralysis than with any other system because you're shortening the curve rather than lengthening it, so there's no stretching of the spinal cord.
>
> I would not say that anterior techniques are for everyone, but in certain cases, including idiopathic patients with a single lumbar or single thoracolumbar curve above 45 degrees, the Zielke would be my first choice. Fifteen years ago, we would have done a Harrington on such a person, but today we feel we'll get better correction, and a better-looking, more mobile patient with Zielke. In addition, we recently completed a careful analysis of one thousand consecutive anterior ap-

proaches done at our institution and found the complication rate was actually less than that of posterior approaches.

That's quite an impressive testimonial. But now let's hear another side of the story from an equally well-known scoliosis surgeon, Dr. Keim:

I do think the anterior approach is warranted in certain selected spinal cases—particularly those where a patient has a severe scoliosis or when patients have very rigid curves that need a release of the soft tissue structures from in front. Of course, people with neurological problems that cause their scoliosis will often benefit from these approaches. However, the anterior approach is not always warranted for routine cases and I doubt very much if the inherent risks of that approach outweigh the advantages of posterior surgery.

I have had a great number of patients whose doctors suggested an anterior approach to the spine and I have operated on them posteriorly. Most of them are eternally grateful, and they are thrilled that they have only had one operation that is from behind. To me, if you can perform an operation on someone with a significant curve and reduce it by almost 50 percent with a posterior approach, why take the risk of an anterior operation only to gain a few more degrees? I really don't think it's worth it.

There are big risks to anterior spine surgery and the complications can be extremely serious. The patient is usually on the operating table longer than he would be with a posterior procedure and because you are working so close to major organs, there is always the possibility of long term complications.

Throughout this chapter, we've seen that there are differing points of view about *all* scoliosis surgeries, and that when it comes to discussions about risks versus benefits, the rhetoric used can create entirely different images of the very same technique. From Dr. Winter, for example, we get a glowing report on the Zielke—it's safe and highly effective. Yet Dr. Keim provides us with a rather frightening scenario of anterior approaches—they're riskier than other procedures, and can result in "significant complications." So whom do you believe?

That's a tough question, one that only you can answer. To my mind, Dr. Winter makes a strong case for the Zielke technique, and I would feel quite confident about proceeding with it if he were the man doing the job. Yet Dr. Keim has an equally convincing argument against it, and if he recommended a posterior approach to me, I'd not hesitate to put my faith in his surgical abilities. I "believe" both of them, because I know that they are highly skilled, experienced scoliosis surgeons whose business it is to make the right decisions for their patients. They're the kind of specialist any person contemplating scoliosis surgery should seek.

I urge you to do your homework before you go ahead with surgery. And that means asking your surgeon pointed questions:

- How many surgeries have you done?

- Which type of technique do you perform most often?

- How many of those do you do each month?

- May I have names and phone numbers of patients on whom you've performed this particular type of surgery?

You should be satisfied with the answers you get, discuss the surgery with your specialist, and understand all the risks that may be involved with your particular condition. If you do all that, you'll be one step closer to a straighter spine and a lifetime of good health.

5

Preparing Yourself for Surgery

If you and your doctor have agreed that you're going to go ahead with surgery, don't expect to be checked into the hospital the very next day. First, he'll do a complete assessment of your spine. You'll have X rays taken in various positions: standing—front and back and to the side—and bending, which will help him determine how flexible your spine really is and how much he'll be able to straighten it. These X rays also provide a graphic record of what your spine was like before surgery and help the doctor determine which procedure will be best for you.

Even if the X rays reveal that you're a good candidate for surgery, you won't be packing your hospital bags just yet. Since scoliosis surgery is rarely performed on an emergency basis, it may be two or three months before you find yourself in the operating room.

For some people, this is an excruciatingly long period of time to wait. They just want to get it over with! Actually, this hiatus is a blessing in disguise because it gives you time to come to terms with the fact that you're really going to have surgery, and to organize your life so that when the big day arrives, there aren't any niggling details hanging over your head or tasks left undone that could interfere with your complete recovery.

CONTACT YOUR INSURANCE CARRIER

Since spine surgery is costly—depending on where you have surgery performed, a one-stage procedure plus a seven-day stay in the hospital can cost between $12,000 and $20,000—the first thing you should do is consult with your insurance agent to see whether the surgery and hospital stay will be covered by your policy. Most insurance companies, such as Blue Cross-Blue Shield, have an 80/20 policy, which means that after you pay your deductible, the company will kick in 80 percent of the surgeon's fee and 80 percent of the cost of the room; you're responsible for the remaining 20 percent. If you belong to a health maintenance organization or HMO, the company may pay 100 percent of the bill.

If you don't have insurance, it's a wise idea to talk with your doctor or his assistant to find out if the hospital provides funds that can be used for those patients with financial difficulties. Failing that, you may want to make arrangements with your bank to take out a loan.

Most insurance companies now require that you get a second opinion; they want to assure themselves that the surgery is required for medical, not cosmetic, reasons. Find out if your insurance policy has this requirement and, if it does, you can ask your orthopedist to refer you to another qualified surgeon.

ORGANIZE PERSONAL DETAILS

Once you've got the financial details in order, you should begin the second phase of presurgical preparations—tying up the loose ends in your personal life. Talk with your teachers or your employer about the length of time you expect to be away. (Your doctor can give you a pretty good estimate of this, based on the type of surgical procedure that will be done, and whether or not you need one operation or two.) Also make sure that these individuals understand that spine surgery is *major* surgery—you won't have the strength or desire to slave over makeup work during your recuperation period. To be sure, there have been people who've had spine surgery and, because they're overachievers or are endowed with big reserves of adrenaline, have managed to overcome postsurgical fatigue and resume the activities of daily life. But for the majority of us, the healthiest way to regain strength after surgery comes from rest, prescribed exercises, well-balanced meals, and support from family and friends, not from sweating over a hot calculator! Whatever you do, don't expend a lot of energy worrying about what you'll be missing while you're away from school or work. It will all be there waiting for you when you return!

If you live alone, or know that you'll be spending the better part of your at-home recuperation by yourself, it's a good idea to arrange to have friends or relatives drop in on you several times a day after you're home from the hospital. No, you're not going to be flat on your back; in fact, you'll probably be up and about for many hours each day. But you may not feel like making your own meals, and you're probably not going to want to slog away at chores such as vacuuming or doing the laundry. In addition, if you have to wear a postsurgical brace, you may find that when you remove it to take a shower, you'll feel dizzy. (Your blood pressure will drop when you remove it.) If that happens, it's comforting to know there's someone just outside the door or down the hall in case you need assistance.

It's also psychologically therapeutic to have someone around during your recovery period. Just having someone to talk with can go a long way toward making you feel better. Many people experience slight depression after surgery, not unlike the "postpartum blues" that strike many women after they've given birth. New mothers feel as if they've lost some control over their lives, or that they'll never get their strength back. The same is true of many people who have any kind of major surgery.

Of course, if you have to wear a postsurgical brace, you may feel frustrated that the "real you" will be under cover for the next several months. I found it particularly aggravating to come to grips with the fact that my snug-fitting clothes would be gathering dust all that time. Had it not been for those daily visits from caring friends and relatives who were willing to listen to me whine every once in a while, I don't think I'd have gotten through my recuperation as well as I did.

About a month before surgery, you will be asked to donate the blood that will be used during your surgery. Hospitals encourage this for several reasons: you're assured of getting your own blood type at the time of surgery; you prevent the danger of hepatitis and the slight risk of complications due to AIDS, the acquired immune deficiency syndrome that has been linked with getting blood transfusions; and, if you're female, by using your own blood, you'll eliminate the risk of developing foreign substances that can interfere with fetal blood should you become pregnant at some time in the future. If, for some reason, you cannot donate your own blood, arrangements can be made for a "designated" donor, a relative or other person whose blood type is identical to yours.

Several weeks in advance, get a good checkup from your local doctor, pediatrician, or internist—someone who knows your health history well. All too often, patients come into the hospital, having spent months waiting for the precious surgical date, only to find that they have high blood pressure, sugar in their urine, or other problems that could have been discovered and treated earlier. "There is such emotional stress getting geared up for surgery," notes Dr. Robert Winter, a specialist at the Minnesota Spine Center, "that it can be catastrophic if the operation has to be canceled for problems like these."

Surgical patients should try to stay in good physical condition as well. Stop smoking if you haven't already. Eat sensibly and keep alcohol consumption to a minimum. And talk with your doctor about whether you need to engage in a fitness or weight-reduction program.

As your hospital date draws near, it's a good idea to make up a checklist of things to bring with you to the hospital. Pack a pair of comfortable slippers without heels, a pair of low-heeled walking shoes, your favorite bathrobe, plus personal grooming items such as your toothbrush, toothpaste, comb, and brush. If you're female and feel you need to bring your make-up, go ahead. But believe me, you won't feel much in the mood to "put on your face." After surgery, I didn't care what I looked like—even though I'd packed enough foundation, blusher, and lipstick for a month of makeovers!

You will be given a hospital gown to wear during the brief period of bed rest after surgery, so you won't need to bring your own pajamas. You may want to pack a comfortable warm-up suit. Once you're out of bed and taking daily walks in the hospital corridors, you may want something that doesn't look "medicinal." One week before surgery, make a special effort to get your rest. "Patients should arrive at the hospital rested, not exhausted," advises Dr. Winter.

Prior to your arrival at the hospital, your doctor will ask you to fill out various forms that the hospital will keep on file, including an *informed consent*. This important document says, in essence, that you and your doctor have discussed the nature of your surgery, as well as its risks and possible complications.

PRE-SURGICAL CHECK-UP

Although you probably won't be checked into the hospital until the *morning* of your surgery, it's likely that you'll spend part or all of the day *before* your surgery at the clinic or hospital out-patient department. There, staff members will perform a pre-admission assessment, which includes a physical exam, X rays, and a variety of tests. For example, the staff will check your blood pressure to make sure your blood will flow properly during surgery; they'll also test your lung capacity to ensure that you're able to inhale and exhale properly. They'll take samples of your blood and urine to make sure you don't have any sort of infection. They'll weigh you and measure your height as well. (If you're having surgery at a hospital located out of state, many of these tests may have been done by your family doctor and forwarded to your surgeon's staff for review.)

During the pre-admission assessment, you and your family will also receive detailed educational information about certain tasks that *must* be performed the night before your surgery. For example, you will learn the technique for administering an enema, a somewhat uncomfortable, but quickly performed procedure that flushes waste from your system. It's an extremely important part of your pre-surgical work-up: the more "cleaned out" you are before surgery, the better you'll feel afterward.

You and your family members also will learn how to do your own pre-surgical "scrub," which involves the use of a special cleanser followed by the application of an antibacterial lotion that stays on your skin and helps to fight off infection. It smells medicinal, sort of like alcohol, but it's also cool and soothing. When rubbed on your back by someone who knows how to give a good backrub, it feels fabulous!

Your pre-surgical staff will answer any questions you may have, including one of the most common: Can I have breakfast the morning of surgery? Their answer will be emphatic: "Nothing to eat or drink after midnight the night before surgery!" (In fact, some spine centers recommend that patients not eat a heavy meal after 7:00 p.m. the night before surgery.) You may, however, brush your teeth in the morning; just don't swallow any water!

THE DAY OF SURGERY

Let's say you're scheduled for a 7:30 a.m. surgery. You will arrive at the hospital that morning around 6:00 a.m. or so. After changing into your hospital gown, you'll be able to spend a little time with parents, friends, or your spouse. (Some patients prefer to spend this time alone. It's perfectly acceptable if you want a little quiet time. Do whatever makes you most comfortable.)

At about 6:30 a.m., you'll ride on a cart to a holding room, where a nurse will give you a sedative to make you drowsy. Most hospitals now do this intraveneously—a needle-like tube, through which fluid is pumped, is inserted into a vein in your arm. Called an I.V., it's slightly uncomfortable at first, but once in place (the tiny needle is secured by adhesive tape), you'll hardly notice it's there. You'll also have to use a catheter, a device that's gently inserted into your urethra so that your urine can pass through it into a container. Sounds awful, I know, but you cannot feel that it's there, and believe me, after surgery, you're not going to want to get up and go to the bathroom!

After you're hooked up to these gizmos, you'll begin to feel the sedative take effect. You'll feel so drowsy so fast that if you try to count backward from ten to one, you'll be asleep by the time you get to six or five.

IN THE OPERATING ROOM

Now you'll be wheeled into the operating room, where a number of activities will be taking place—all without your knowing it, of course! First, you'll be turned over on your stomach (if you are having a posterior procedure), and positioned on four "posters" that prop you up beneath your chest and hips so that you have plenty of breathing room. Your head will rest on a pillow, and your arms and legs will be positioned on other soft supports. You'll also be hooked up to two or three devices: one that supervises your heart during surgery; another that monitors the nerve endings of your spinal cord, although this is not used in every case; and an instrument that can replace blood while the surgeon operates. Once these are in place, your anesthesiologist, who will sit by you during the entire operation, will place a breathing tube into your mouth or nose, through which you'll breathe in the *anesthetic,* the sweet-smelling gas that will keep you asleep and oblivious to pain.

At many hospitals, doctors who perform scoliosis surgery will use the *Stagnara Wake-up test,* a technique used to monitor the spinal cord. During the operation, the patient is briefly brought to an appropriate level of consciousness and asked to wiggle his or her toes. Most patients will not remember that the wake-up test was performed.

Now the surgical team, having scrubbed up and donned their surgical gowns and masks, is ready to begin. Using a scalpel, your surgeon will make a *midline incision,* drawn in a straight line despite the fact your back is curved. The length of the incision will depend, of course, upon the length of your curve(s). The surgeon and his team will then spend the next three to four hours straightening your curve, using one of the several techniques commonly used today. As you learned in Chapter 4, he'll fasten various rods and/or wires to your vertebrae, and place small chips of bone along your newly straightened spine that will fuse to it and create a solid mass of bone. By the time your spine heals, the rods and/or wires no longer serve any function, but remain inside you for the rest of your life. To take them out would mean another surgery and who would want that?

After the surgeon is satisfied that all the instrumentation is securely in place, he'll close up most of the incision with *dissolvable sutures,* tiny threads that eliminate the "railroad track" sort of scar. (In fact, by the time you heal, your scar will be just a fine line. Mine is hardly visible, unless you're really looking for it.) In the small open space along the incision, the surgeon will insert a *hemovac tube,* which helps drain out excess body fluid and blood that may accumulate.

Now the surgical team will remove the heart monitor and blood transfusion device, then gently turn you on your back. A nurse will wheel you (and your I.V. and, if necessary, the spinal cord monitor) to a postanesthesia care unit, where you'll spend the next three or four hours. You'll still be in a deep sleep, however, so you won't be aware that nurses are still monitoring your blood pressure and taking X rays of your spine. In addition, your I.V. will now be pumping antibiotics into your system; this is necessary so that your body can fight off any infection that might occur.

AFTER SURGERY

Once you pass post-operative inspection, you'll be taken to an intensive care or special scoliosis unit of the hospital. You'll spend about forty-eight hours here, during which time your hemovac tube, catheter, and any remaining monitoring devices will be removed. Because the anesthesia will begin to wear off now, this is a time of complete bed rest—you'll be flat on your back and asked not to raise your head beyond 30 degrees so that you don't put any pressure on your spine. Every two hours or so, however, two nurses will "log roll" your body. Using a bedsheet for leverage, they'll gently roll your body to one side, then the other. This keeps you from getting bed sores, and also keeps you from getting stiff.

Because your lungs were "relaxed" during surgery, they now need to get a little exercise, so every four hours or so you'll be asked to blow into an *inspirometer* for as long as you're able. This procedure also helps push out any mucus that might have accumulated during surgery, a situation that can sometimes lead to pneumonia. Many people find these "blow bottle" exercises extremely difficult; they're just so tired and weak that they don't want to do much besides rest. But do your best to puff away as often as you're asked to. Once you put your mind to it, you'll be surprised to learn how much lung power you really have!

During these two days of post-op observation, you'll be allowed to have visitors, but only for a few minutes at a time. Of course, most nurses are pretty flexible about extending visits, but believe me, you're probably not going to feel much like schmoozing with parents or pals for more than ten or fifteen minutes. You're still going to feel groggy; it can take anywhere from twenty-four to forty-eight hours to completely recover from the anesthesia.

On day three, if not earlier, you'll be moved to a special section of the hospital reserved for scoliosis patients. You'll still have the antibiotic I.V. attached to your arm, but your nurse will have added a pain medication to the fluid. Much as I'd like to say that scoliosis surgery doesn't hurt, I have to be honest. It does hurt. But thanks to the pain medication, these periods of discomfort can be managed.

Later in the day, your I.V. will be removed, but you can always ask for an occasional pain pill if you need it. Your appetite will have returned a little, and you'll be able to eat gelatin, soup, and milk. You'll also begin taking iron tablets, which will keep your blood and bones strong and healthy. In some cases, though, iron supplements can cause constipation, so you may have to take a mild laxative.

Depending upon the type of surgery you've had, you may be up and walking within forty-eight hours or so after surgery. This quick recovery time absolutely amazes me—when I had my first surgery back in 1970, my surgeon recommended I spend nearly two weeks afterward flat on my back! You'll probably feel weak and a little wobbly when you first get out of bed; that's perfectly natural, and nothing to worry about—you'll be getting stronger with each passing day. These first walks are never long and arduous—just five or ten minutes up and down the hallway. And in some ways they're fun; you're taking the first steps toward a successful recovery, and the new friends you've made in the hospital will be cheering you on!

On the fourth day after surgery, you'll be ready to be fitted for a brace *if you've had the type of surgery that requires one.* The procedure, which involves the creation of a plaster impression of your body, is usually performed at your bedside. Depending upon your age and how quickly your fusion heals, you'll wear your postsurgical brace, made of plastic or fiber glass, which resembles a low-profile brace (see Chapter 3, "Nonsurgical Treatments"), for approximately four to six months. During the final days of your hospital stay—five to seven days for a single-stage procedure—you'll continue blending rest with daily walks to help build up your strength.

If you're wearing a brace, you may find that relatively simple tasks—such as bending over to pick something up, dressing yourself, or walking up and down stairs—aren't as easy to do as they used to be. A physical therapist will be available to help you practice doing these things in the brace. For example, to avoid the tendency to lean back in your brace while navigating on stairs, your therapist will teach you how to push yourself forward so you don't lose your balance. You'll also learn how to bend at the knees when you have to retrieve something from the floor.

For those who will be wearing a brace, the simple act of dressing can be a formidable task, but this problem too can be overcome. For example, putting on shoes and stockings is easy to do if you bring up each ankle and rest it on the opposite knee. Donning a skirt or a pair of slacks can also be accomplished without much of a struggle—you place the garment on your bed, then lie down and slither your way into it. Don't worry if you feel clumsy for the first few weeks after surgery; you'll get more adept at dressing yourself and doing other tasks as you continue to regain your strength.

RECUPERATING AT HOME

For the first four to six weeks after surgery, you should get as much rest as you need, but also increase the walking exercises. They are essential to the healing process. In fact, studies have shown that the more physical conditioning you get after surgery, the faster you heal. But remember, walking is best; refrain from those "no pain/ no gain" workouts! Also avoid excessive bending and twisting for any reason, and do not lift heavy objects. Keep in mind that it takes four to six months for an adolescent's fusion to heal, and six to twelve months for an adult's.

Because the body uses a lot of energy to heal itself, patients should increase their caloric intake during the recuperative period, or longer if their doctor advises. Don't worry about becoming a "blimp"; your body will be burning off the extra calories while it's mending.

What about sexual activity during the recuperative period? Although you should talk with your doctor about your particular condition and how sex might affect it, generally speaking, it's perfectly all right to engage in sexual intercourse while you're recuperating—as long as you're using an effective means of birth control. According to Dr. Winter: "With modern internal fixation techniques and good postoperative support, sexual activity can continue and there is no reason to avoid it for fear of upsetting the operative procedures. Sometimes the margin of the brace can be irritating to the partner; in these cases, the edges can be padded. Acrobatic positions during intercourse should be avoided. The person who has had the surgery should, in most circumstances, take the less-active role during intercourse." And, remember, if you've been instructed to wear a postoperative brace, make sure you keep it on during sexual activity.

About two weeks after surgery, adolescents usually can return to school, whereas adults may need anywhere from four to eight weeks or more to gain enough strength to return to work. In most cases, youngsters and adults can resume activities that were a part of life before surgery, except for rough contact sports such as football. With your doctor's permission, you may be able to swim (without the brace if you have one) for a couple of hours a week. Each scoliosis case is different, so make sure you talk with your doctor before engaging in any sports activities.

About four to six weeks after surgery, you'll return to the clinic or hospital for X rays. These will show your doctor (and you—if you want to see them) that your instrumentation is firmly in place and doing its job of correcting your curve. You'll return several months later for more X rays, at which time those tiny bone chips used for grafting should have knitted together to form a solid bone mass. If they have, your doctor will probably give you permission to remove the brace—if one was required—for several hours each day so that you can swim, or do other types of exercises that he'll prescribe. He'll also be able to give you a rough idea of when you can remove the brace forever!

By the time you're free of the brace, you'll be back to normal. You'll be as active as ever, and you'll feel better than you ever did before surgery. Because your curve has been straightened out, you'll be taller now—anywhere from one to four inches or more! Your clothes will fit better, too: shoulders, waistlines, and hems will be straighter, and if you had a rib hump before surgery, you can expect that it will be less noticeable or that it's disappeared altogether!

6

What Patients Say About Spine Surgery

Whenever I meet someone who is faced with the prospect of having spine surgery, I can usually predict that the individual will ask one or more of the following questions: "What's it like to have surgery?" "Does it hurt?" "How will I feel afterward?" "Will I be glad I had it done, or will I regret it?"

Throughout this chapter, you'll get answers to those and other questions, because you'll meet youngsters and adults who've had operations to correct their scoliosis and who can tell you about their surgical experience in their own words.

A POSITIVE ATTITUDE ENSURED SUCCESS

Randy Peterson is one of many people who wish they'd had scoliosis surgery a lot sooner than they did. Although he was diagnosed as having scoliosis at the age of thirteen, it was not until 1986, when he turned twenty-two, that he finally checked into the hospital to have it corrected. Unlike many people I interviewed, Randy did not ignore his curve during those intervening years. Far from it! He wore a Milwaukee brace, night and day, for five whole years—but unfortunately, as sometimes happens, his stubborn curve refused to respond to it.

"In seventh grade, when my mom and I noticed that my rib cage was twisted a little, we went to our family doctor. He took X rays, and we learned that I had a slight curve of about 10 degrees. He said it probably was nothing to worry about, but suggested we see a doctor at a scoliosis clinic, just to be on the safe side. By the time we got around to making the appointment—about two months later—my curve had progressed to 25 degrees. It was just racing out of control! I wasn't in any kind of pain, and my rib cage didn't really look worse, but we couldn't ignore what the X rays were saying.

"So they put me in a Milwaukee brace, neck ring and all. Needless to say, my reaction was *very* negative. I didn't want to go back to school, and I had a lot of trouble getting clothing to fit over it. No matter how much padding there is on braces, they just eat up your clothes. I never bought a decent shirt the whole time I had to wear my brace.

"I wore that thing twenty-three hours a day, every day, but each time I went back for a checkup, my curve was 5 to 10 degrees worse. By the time I reached twelfth grade, it had progressed into the high 40s. But because of my age, the doctors felt that I'd matured enough so that it would slow down or stop at that point. So they finally took me out of the brace, and we all agreed that I'd keep coming back for checkups from time to time.

"I kept going back to the clinic while I was in college and, sure enough, it got worse. Finally, when the curve had reached 62 degrees, the doctors told me that I couldn't put off surgery any longer. They were worried that the curve might cause some spinal cord damage. And by now, my body had changed quite a bit—although I didn't have a rib hump, my chest and shoulders were so uneven, it looked like my body was twisted half over to the other side.

"My first reaction was, 'Well, I knew this was coming,' because it had kept on getting worse over the last four or five years. But my second reaction was one of bitterness—why did I have to spend all those years in the brace when it didn't seem to have done me a whole heck of a lot of good?

"I was pretty frustrated about it, because I've also had a lot of medical problems ever since I was little—none of them little picky things, either. I was born with a cleft lip and cleft palate, and had to have major surgery to correct those. And since those problems caused a severe underbite, and because my teeth were all over the place in my mouth, I had to have more surgery to move my front jaw out about an inch and a half, then had to have my mouth wired shut for a month. By themselves, those surgeries wouldn't have been so bad, but I was in the Milwaukee brace at the time I had them done! Still, I'm a pretty tough bird most of the time, and I really have never let that kind of crap get me down. But believe me, there have been days when I've felt, 'God, just to be average!'

"Maybe because I'd gone through other types of surgery, I wasn't that upset about having scoliosis surgery. Of course, I was going through finals week at college, so I didn't really have much time to think about it.

"The night before I had surgery, the doctor came in and explained that he was going to do a Cotrel-Dubousset technique on me—he'd fuse eight of my vertebrae and then put in two rods with wires. He did say he might wind up doing something different once he got in there because they often don't know for sure which technique to use until they actually see your spine. But at that point, he was pretty sure he'd do the C-D, and that meant I probably wouldn't have to wear a brace after surgery. As a person who'd already spent five years cooped up in a brace, I was relieved to hear this—in fact, that's probably the only reason I didn't cut out of the hospital and go home that night! I'd seriously considered just sneaking out and getting on a bus and going home—nobody would have known where to find me!

"I really got a lot of psychological support from the nurses. Many of them had had scoliosis surgery themselves. When I asked one of them, who had become pregnant many months after her surgery, whether having a steel rod in her back was hard on her, she said, 'No, I hardly notice it at all.' Just hearing that made me feel a whole lot better.

"I wasn't too nervous the night before surgery, but in the morning, that was a different story. I was real nervous then. But my mom and dad were there, and that helped a lot. Both of them have had surgery for disc problems, so we all talked about our feelings. It was nice to know that they could personally understand what I was going through.

"I wasn't too worried about the pain after surgery—I've done a lot of hurting in one way or another in my life. But when the anesthesia wore off, it felt as if a Mack truck had run over my back—literally! Let me tell you, I don't cry very often, but that was quite a night! I was only in really bad pain for about a half an hour, though, because they gave me medication. Don't get me wrong. It still hurt, but it wasn't unbearable.

"I'm the kind of person who doesn't let things slow me down, so the day after surgery, I was out of bed walking around. I got out of the hospital about seven days later and didn't have much trouble at all. I did a lot of sleeping and lying around, but I never got depressed—I don't let stuff like that get me down too much.

"About three and a half weeks after surgery, I was back into the swing of things. I had to take it a little easy at school—I couldn't carry the twenty pounds of books I used to lug around with me— and I did get tired a lot. But overall, surgery hasn't slowed me down hardly at all.

"Although my curve was corrected to about 30 degrees, I'm still a little crooked, but basically, I'm much better. My shoulders are much more even now, and so is my chest. And even though I didn't have any cardiopulmonary problems, I think I'm breathing better now. To me, the surgery was well worth it.

"Anybody who's going to have surgery needs to 'hang tough,' I think. It'll be rough for a while, but in the long run, it's better to go through with it because you can take all the pain in a week's time, and then not have the problems for the rest of your life. Or you can do nothing and have real serious problems forever. The aftereffects of surgery can be hard to live with, but the only thing that can really slow you down is your own attitude about it. If you've got a good, positive attitude about surgery, it really doesn't slow you down much at all."

A FANTASTIC SHAPE

Although Maria Halpin, now fifty-two, knew she had scoliosis at the age of thirteen, she spent many years ignoring her curve until, around 1980, it had progressed to 84 degrees. By that time, although her lumbar curve was not terribly noticeable—she could conceal it with the "right" clothes—there was no ignoring the pain. Still, it was not until 1984 that she finally had surgery and, as you'll see, the anxiety she suffered in the intervening years was more than most people deal with in a lifetime. Happily for Maria, however, the ordeal was worth it.

"I suffered for many years from the scoliosis in my back, but I really didn't know anything could be done about it. I kept fooling myself that it wasn't getting worse. I kept eliminating activities from my life so that I'd have less pain and sometimes I could convince myself that the pain had decreased, but it really hadn't—I was just doing a lot less.

"All the doctors I went to in America and in Germany, where I once lived, said nothing could be done for me. No one ever mentioned that surgery was available. I'm amazed that no doctor ever even hinted to me about it. So I kept looking around for books and articles on the subject, and finally, in a book about general health, I found a section about scoliosis, and that's the first time I ever knew there was such a thing as Harrington rod surgery.

"That gave me a little hope, so I went to an orthopedic surgeon in Atlanta to see whether anything could be done. I told him I had a lot of pain, and he took an X ray of my spine that showed my curve was 84 degrees. He said he couldn't do a thing except give me exercises to do! I couldn't believe it! I said to him, 'I have so much pain and you tell me there is nothing you can do?' As I said this, he was instructing his nurse to give me information about the exercises and was about to leave the room when I said, 'What about surgery and the Harrington rod?'

"His eyes lit up and he said, 'You mean you'd be interested in something like that?' I said that I would, and he gave me the name of a spine specialist.

"When I met with the new surgeon, I wasn't convinced that I should have the surgery. It seemed scary and frightening to me, and the surgeon seemed cold and unfeeling toward me. I didn't trust him, didn't get a good feeling about him, so I decided that I would just continue to try and live with the pain.

"That didn't work, and I eventually found another surgeon. He took X rays of my spine and told me that I must have surgery and that I should not wait any longer. But then he showed me an X ray of another patient who had surgery and it looked terrible and shocking to me. I thought, 'No, I'll never have this done to me.' He did, however, give me the name of another orthopedist. I agreed to meet with him, but I knew in my heart I probably couldn't go through with it.

"When I met the new doctor, he took X rays of my spine. My curve had progressed to 87 degrees. Of course, he recommended that I have surgery, and by now I knew he was right. The whole atmosphere at the center was good and comforting—I knew it was the right place.

"At first, I thought I'd only have to have one surgery. But after doing a lot of tests, the doctor told me that because many of my discs were destroyed because of scoliosis, he'd have to do two surgeries—a Zielke first and then a Luque—and fuse my spine all the way down to my hips! That really scared me, but he said it wouldn't make much difference in my life, that I could still do all the same things I'd done before. It took me a while to accept this, but I knew I would be in good hands. Thankfully, I had done a lot of research beforehand—all that information helped me judge for myself.

"The night before surgery, I felt very positive. I blocked out any fearful thoughts from my mind. I had made up my mind that this was it. I knew my surgeon was an expert, and the rest would be up to Somebody Up There. Of course, my husband spent a lot of time with me at the hospital. He was very supportive and that helped a lot. But I knew most of it was up to me.

"After the first surgery, I felt very much at peace and that everything was going to be just fine. I did have some pain, but a different kind than I had felt before. Your body is just in an upheaval after surgery, but luckily, I was mentally prepared for it so it wasn't that bad. I think you get mentally strong when you know you're going to have surgery. I got through the first surgery fine, so I believed the second one would be all right, too.

"After the first surgery, I wasn't allowed to get out of bed before having the second one. But after I had the Luque, I was out of bed in four days. It was absolutely scary the first time I got up, but I did it and after that it just got easier and easier.

"Ten days after the final surgery, I left the hospital to go back home. I felt fine, but I was afraid of having to take all those taxis to and from the airport, and to get on the plane. It was quite an undertaking, but luckily, I was able to lie down in the plane and rest, and I continued taking my pain pills. I did much better than I ever imagined!

"When I got home, I kept thinking that the pain would never stop. When I would lie down, I felt good, but as soon as I'd get up, I got this indescribable pain—sort of like somebody pressing a big shoe in your back. But then, all of a sudden, the pain was just gone. It didn't fade away, it just disappeared. And within six weeks after the last surgery, I felt like my old self again. I continued wearing my brace for nine months, though I took it off for a while each day so that I could take a shower. And I also did a lot of walking—two miles a day!

"My surgeon was right. I can do everything I did before, but now, instead of bending at the waist, I bend at the hips and come down with my knees a bit if I have to pick something up. It is no problem whatsoever, and I don't even notice it anymore.

"I don't know how much improved my curve is in degrees and I didn't even ask. I'm not interested! I think I look perfectly straight compared to what I was before. And my scars are very nice—one starts on the side of my navel and goes around my hip upward to the back near my lower rib and the other is in the middle of my back. They both look good. I'm even going to a public swimming pool in a bathing suit—and that's something I would have never done before!

"If I had known in 1980 what I know now, I'd have gone for surgery right away. It helps a lot to do your research, call anybody you can, read everything you can, and inform yourself before you go ahead with surgery. Then you make up your mind. I'm glad I did, because I'm in such fantastic shape now!"

COMPLICATED BUT WORTH IT

Fifty-two-year-old Jane Williams (not her real name) battled scoliosis nearly all her life. Diagnosed as having idiopathic scoliosis at the age of six, she spent the next several years wearing a corset and doing a variety of exercises. She was told these remedies would correct her curvature, but they didn't, and by the time she turned eleven, her curve had progressed to nearly 100 degrees. Not only did her S-shaped curvature create a huge rib hump on her back, it also squeezed her lungs so that her breathing capacity was only 35 percent. Since that time, Jane has had four spine surgeries to correct her scoliosis, each one fraught with complications. But despite all the problems, she believes the surgeries were worth it. Today, when she looks in the mirror, she still remarks, "I can't believe it's me!"

Jane says, "Before I had my first two surgeries—spinal fusions done two weeks apart—I spent three months in the hospital bound up in a turnbuckle cast that covered most of my head and enveloped my body down to my knees. The cast was supposed to stretch me out a bit before I had the fusions. My parents and I went along with this because we believed that all these procedures would eventually get rid of my rib hump. But apparently we misunderstood the doctors—they don't always word things too well—because even after the surgeries, my hump was still there. The doctors told me there was no way of getting rid of it after all. As you can imagine, I was absolutely devastated!

"Even though the fusions reduced my curve to 89 degrees, and the doctor told me my back was strong enough that I could be a hog carrier and that everything would be just fine, that didn't turn out to be true. Though I carried on with my life for many years, by the time I reached menopause, I started having respiratory problems. I coughed all the time and was so short of breath that just walking from the parking lot to the hospital where I worked left me gasping. So I had X rays taken and learned that, despite the fusions, my curve had increased to 110 degrees!

"Eventually, I went to another hospital and the doctor said he could fix my spine by doing two more surgeries—an anterior and a posterior. I was frightened, but I knew I had to do something. I didn't want to spend the rest of my life as a respiratory cripple.

"I had to wait for three months before the hospital could take me, and even in that short period of time, my curve increased from 110 to 116 degrees. But when I checked into the hospital in January 1986, I was full of high hopes and not the least bit frightened. Three people who had had the same type of surgeries had written to me and said they were feeling and looking great, and I also prayed a lot and felt that I received signs that said, 'Go ahead with the surgery . . . it'll be great!'

"After the first surgery, well, you name the complication and I had it. I developed a pulmonary embolism, a blood clot on the lung. When you reach my age and you have lung complications to begin with on top of the surgery, it's no wonder this happened. Then I developed a bladder infection and a kidney stone (a problem I'd had before), and from all the medications I was taking, the iron pills and pain pills, I developed gastritis. My stomach blew up like I was six or seven months' pregnant. Needless to say, they had to postpone the second surgery for a few weeks until all those problems cleared up.

"I was scared to go back for the second procedure, but as I've always said, 'If you're swimming and reach the middle of the lake, you have to keep on going to get to the other side.' So of course I went ahead with it. But I was miserable for quite a while afterward. I was worried that I'd develop another clot (but didn't), and I was in quite a lot of pain. I hated even being touched!

"My curve is now down to 85 degrees, and even though I still tire pretty easily and am not too crazy about having to wear this brace, I think I look terrific and I'm breathing very well.

"When I used to look at myself from the front, I looked a little dumpy. One of my breasts looked crooked, and so were my shoulders—I looked like a tube of toothpaste that had been squeezed together, with a great big hump on the back of it. But now that I've straightened out, I just can't believe it's me! Even friends who used to say that they never noticed my hump think I look wonderful now, even though I have the brace on!

"For me, the surgeries were hell, but they were short-lived. If you compare that to a lifetime, it's worth it. What're a few months compared to years of agony that keeps getting worse? Even with all the complications, if I had it to do over again, I would. What the doctors did for me was unbelievable!"

A GOOD MIND SET HELPS

Lisa Gervais, twenty-five, is a "tough cookie" by just about anyone's standards. Lisa ignored the protests of her worried parents and scheduled herself for spine surgery in November 1985. She claims the experience never caused her a bit of pain, and attributes her phenomenal recovery to her belief in "mind over matter."

"When I was thirteen, my school doctor noticed a curve in my back and sent notes with me to take home to my mother. But because I was heavily into gymnastics and didn't want anything to ruin that, I threw the notes in the garbage. I knew somebody who had scoliosis and she had to wear a brace—I didn't want to have to do that! The thought of having to wear a brace really scared me.

"Nobody in my family knew there was anything wrong, and because I wasn't feeling any pain or having any other symptoms, I just went through high school with sort of a 'la-di-da' attitude. I didn't notice that my body was curving at all, so I figured that there really wasn't anything wrong.

"After I graduated and got a full-time job and had to sit at a desk all day long, it finally hit me. I started having a lot of pain in the middle of my back and in my shoulder blades. I still looked okay, but I had the pain, so I went to see an orthopedist. He took X rays and said my curve was about 42 degrees. But because I was seventeen and almost full-grown, he didn't recommend a brace. He said it probably wouldn't do me much good, and suggested that we just watch it to see if it would progress.

"I wasn't upset at that point, knowing how much worse it had gotten. I had made my choice earlier, by throwing away all those notes from the school doctor, and now I knew that I was going to have to live with it.

"About a year later, I went to a specialist who said he could operate on me. But because I wasn't having any trouble breathing and he said the curve wasn't that bad, we decided we'd just wait a while longer to see if it got worse.

"When I turned nineteen, my curve seemed to get a lot worse. I couldn't breathe properly, and I'd get stuck in one position from sitting all day at work. To get relief from the pain, I'd have to come home every night and lie flat on my back. So I started thinking about surgery again, but my parents were very scared of the idea and didn't want me to have it done, so I waited two more years before I saw a specialist again.

"By the time I was twenty-one, my hips were starting to hurt, and I felt as if I was shrinking. I just didn't feel good anymore. I couldn't bend the way I did before, my waist was all bunched up, and my clothes were tight around one shoulder. But I knew some people who'd had scoliosis surgery—people with curves a lot worse than mine—and they'd come through it just fine. So I made an appointment with an orthopedic surgeon.

"After he looked at my X ray, which showed my curve had progressed to 45 degrees, he told me I should have the operation. I was relieved when he said that, because I was going to ask him if I could have the surgery even if he didn't feel I needed it yet. I knew then that it would probably keep progressing unless I did something about it, and I just figured, 'Why not have it done now, while you're still young?' I really wanted to have it done, because I was freaked out because I thought I was shrinking.

"A week before the surgery I checked into the hospital and they put a plaster cast on me to stretch me out a bit. I was feeling really good about it, because I knew that from then on I was going to look and feel better.

"I was never nervous about the surgery. Not one bit. That's because I had a tremendous amount of confidence in my doctor. When he explained the surgery to me, which involved a Harrington rod, he talked about it like it was an afternoon tea party for him, and I figured if it was like that for him, then I had nothing to fear. And the man has done so many operations, so I figured there was no reason for me to get upset.

"When I woke up after surgery, I didn't feel any pain at all. Honestly, it didn't hurt, though my doctor tells me I'm an exception to the rule. Maybe that's because I had worked out on weights for two years before the surgery—I was in really good physical condition. And afterward, I was very mobile; I could move from side to side, and I even handled my own bed pan all by myself.

"Of course, I had a good mind-set. I was determined to have a good recovery, and I didn't ever let myself think I was unhealthy because I'm not unhealthy—I was just apparently born with a curvature of the spine, and that doesn't mean I'm unhealthy.

"Although I wasn't supposed to, I got up out of bed the second day after surgery. I just had to go to the bathroom, and I was real tired of using that bed pan. So I got the nurses to help me to the bathroom, and I didn't feel faint or anything.

"By the seventh day after surgery, I'd gotten my brace and was taking twenty-minute walks on my own. As a matter of fact, before the nurse came into the room to take me down to the main floor so I could go home, I'd taken a shower and gotten dressed by myself.

"Once I got home, about the only problem I had was getting out of deep, cushiony chairs. And because I had to wear a brace, my bed didn't feel too comfortable, and I often felt really warm during the night. But I never needed any help getting dressed, I never took any pain pills, and I didn't take one nap.

"Today I can do everything that I did before. I'm just as flexible as ever, and I can still lift things, as long as I do it properly. And I think I look much better. My waist is a lot longer and slenderer than it was, and I got an inch and a half taller. From the side, my rear end and lower back look a little flatter than they used to because they had to fuse a little way down into my lumbar spine, and I can't say that I like the look. ['Flat back syndrome' has been known to occur in patients whose lumbar areas were fused with a single Harrington rod. The syndrome can cause low back pain years after the surgery, and can produce fatigue and nagging discomfort. Surgeons who specialize in reconstructive surgery have developed techniques to correct this problem.] But I'm still much better than I was before.

"I know I made the right choice. I didn't have any problems at all, and that's because 50 percent of it was me having a good mental attitude and being strong and in good condition. The other 50 percent is that my doctor was so wonderful and good at what he does.

"To me, the surgery did not hurt. I was not uncomfortable, and I really mean that. But it's all in your mental attitude—I believe my mind has total control over everything I do and feel. Sure, you can make it miserable—my roommate in the hospital showed me that. She wasn't happy with anything or comfortable with anything. But she didn't try to be happy or comfortable, she didn't try to feel better. She just lay there in her misery, and she loved it! She didn't like the postsurgical brace, but she didn't even try to like it, so that made it even worse. She had a very bad time of it, but I think it's because she had a bad attitude to begin with.

"To me, the surgery was easy, though I know not everybody feels that way. I was lucky. In two weeks, I was out of there and felt great! I had just made up my mind that it was going to be fine, and it really was!"

QUICK RECOVERY, "WONDERFUL" RESULTS

Like many adults who have scoliosis, Carolee McGinley, fifty-five, knew something was wrong at an early age—in her case, at fourteen. But because she developed a curvature at a time when doctors were not particularly well-informed about scoliosis, she "learned to live with it" for many years. Luckily, however, she never gave up trying to find a surgeon who'd be willing to operate and today this mother of three grown children is happy, healthy, and as she puts it, "straightened out."

Carolee says, "My mother first spotted my scoliosis in 1948. I was dressed up to be in a wedding, and she noticed that the buttons weren't straight and that my shoulders were off. Because this was the era of the polio epidemic, when we went to a doctor shortly thereafter, he said he thought it might be caused by polio (though we're really not sure about that, even today). But since he didn't know how to prevent it from getting worse, he said the best thing to do was rest, and he wouldn't allow me to participate in any high school activities such as gym class.

"Eventually, I found another doctor who sent me to a workshop for polio victims at the Sister Kenney Institute. I went there three times a week, where they'd hang my body from the ceiling from ropes, which was supposed to keep the curve flexible and to keep it from getting worse.

"I thought it was helping, but a few years later, when I had to go into the hospital to have my appendix removed, a doctor noticed the curve and said, 'Gee, you really should have surgery for that.' But when my parents called my family doctor and told him that, he advised against it, saying that if I had surgery, I'd end up in a wheelchair. He didn't believe spine surgery was perfected enough in those days, and he thought it would be too risky. As for my parents, well, in those days, parents didn't really want to own up to their children's problems. Mine sent me to modeling school— they just thought scoliosis was something that would go away. As a result, I pretty much had to figure out what to do on my own.

"By the time I was thirty-eight, I was in terrible pain all the time. After each pregnancy, I gained about sixty pounds, and having to carry my children around just seemed to throw me off. My curve was getting worse, but I still couldn't find a doctor who'd do the surgery—they all thought I was too old and I suppose they were worried about malpractice, too. I got really discouraged. 'I guess I waited too long,' I'd say to my husband. 'Nobody's going to operate on a grandma.'

"Finally, after a lot of probing, I found a new doctor who took X rays of my spine. The curve was about 70 degrees, and he said he couldn't see that there'd be any reason in the world why I couldn't have surgery. I was elated. I was primed for it. And I made an appointment for the surgery. But so many people kept telling me I was nuts to go through with such a serious surgery, I eventually changed my mind and canceled it. I just figured I could live with the pain.

"I couldn't. The pain got really bad—sort of a burning sensation in my back and a numbness in my legs. So I went back to the doctor and he said he'd operate on me and put in a Harrington rod to straighten me out. I'd done a lot of research, though, and knew that sometimes a lumbar curve like mine can wind up looking unnaturally flat when a Harrington rod is inserted, and that it might tilt my body forward. So I decided to get a second opinion. What did I have to lose?

"The doctor told me it would be better for my particular curve to have two operations—an anterior and a posterior with Luque wires. So I decided to go ahead with it, and in January I checked into the hospital.

"I had a lot of nightmares about the surgeries. I always imagined that I'd wake up a paraplegic or something. I just kept thinking, 'I'm bad now, but am I going to be worse off afterward?'

"I can't say I had any real pain after the first surgery. I was so heavily sedated, I can't really remember. But to me, the hardest part of the two-stage procedure is the psychological part, knowing that after you've made it through the first one, you've got to get ready for a second one. I felt as if I was going to crumble, and I wouldn't wish that feeling on anyone.

"But there was a chaplain in the hospital who came to see me every day. He was marvelous! One of the most supportive men I think I've ever met. He was there just for me, and made me feel as though everything was going to be wonderful. That was a big help, because my husband couldn't be there the entire time. It was nice to know that if you cried, you wouldn't have to cry alone.

"Everything went fine with both surgeries and three weeks later, I got fitted for my brace and was allowed to go home. But the recuperation period was tough because I was home alone most of the time. I did hire a day-care person to come in to make the beds each day, and occasionally an RN stopped by to see how I was doing, but I mostly had to do everything myself. After the second week at home, in fact, I did all my own cooking and practically all of the cleaning.

"I didn't have that much pain once I got home. Of course, the surgery is sort of like having a baby—you forget the pain very soon! I did feel a burning sensation where they did the fusion, but I just took a couple of extra-strength Tylenol and that took care of the problem.

"I think I'm a fast healer. I bounced back very quickly after surgery. After just three and a half months, I was doing all the lawn work and gardening—even trimming all the shrubbery with electric shears. And now, just five months after surgery, I'm in the process of stripping off all our wallpaper so that I can repaint the walls!

"Now that my curve is about 35 degrees—half of what it used to be—I can wear dresses with a waistline and no one knows that I ever had scoliosis. I used to be so ashamed, having to wear dresses that were too big for me in order to hide my curve. The first time I went out to buy a dress after surgery was the most wonderful experience in the world—I didn't have to hide in the fitting room!

"Today I think my overall appearance is great, but because they had to fuse the lower part of my spine, I don't think my gait is as natural as it used to be. When I walk slowly, like when you're walking up an aisle, I notice that I'm a little off-balance. I feel stiffer, and can't move the way I did before. And even though the doctors told me this before surgery, it still bothers me. It's something you just have to get used to.

"Every so often, someone will ask me whether or not they should have surgery. If a person has the choice to have the surgery done early in life, I'd say go for it!"

FAMILY AND FRIENDS PROVIDE
INVALUABLE SUPPORT

Laney Moss, seventeen, is one of many youngsters who were wise
enough to "go for" surgery at an early age. But first, she tried
everything she could to avoid it.

"When I went for my yearly checkup at thirteen, my doctor
didn't notice that I had a curvature. But a month later, my gymnastics coach pointed it out. I wasn't all that surprised, because
when I used to do handsprings or walkovers, I'd get these sharp
pains in my back. I kind of thought something might be wrong.

"So we went to an orthopedist and found out that I had a 28-
degree curve. I had to wear a Boston brace—which I named
Oscar—for about a year. I never took it off, except for half an hour
every day to take a shower. And I did lots of exercises, too, even
while I was wearing it. After about six months, Oscar had reduced
the size of my curve. But when I had X rays taken at the end of the
year, my curve was getting close to 40 degrees. By then, my
shoulder jutted out toward the front about three inches, and I
always had to stand in a certain way to try to look straight. The
doctor said we'd have to start thinking about surgery.

"Everybody told me it was up to me to decide, but I said, 'It's
not up to me, because there's nothing I personally can do about it.'
I just had to face it, because I didn't want my curve to get any
worse.

"I had the surgery in September 1985. I didn't really know what
the doctors were going to do to me, but the night before, they
showed a film that explained more about it. I started getting
worried, but both my parents were there, and a bunch of friends
called to say good luck, so it wasn't that bad. If my parents hadn't
been there, it would have been bad, I think, because it can be scary
and it helps to have someone to talk to.

"I wasn't scared the morning of the surgery, except when they
were taking me down to the operating room and at one point they
told my parents they couldn't walk with me any farther. Then I
started crying, but I really don't know what I was afraid of. I don't
like shots—I'm a big baby when it comes to stuff like that. I think I
got scared because I didn't know what was going to happen. So I
just kept asking the doctors, 'You're not going to hurt me, are

you?' They all said no, they wouldn't hurt me. And then someone gave me a shot to put me to sleep, and I don't remember a thing until I got to my regular hospital room.

"The doctors had told me that I'd hurt afterward and they were right. After surgery [which involved a Harrington rod affixed with wires], I was in a lot of pain. Like a throbbing from below my butt up to my neck. But they do give you medicine and that makes you feel better.

"It took quite a while to get my strength back. For five or six days after surgery, I just ate ice chips and was real weak. I was starving, but once I got my food, I didn't feel like eating it. My stomach was upset, and I couldn't go to the bathroom. So when they wheeled me down to get the plaster mold fitted for my brace, my legs were shaking and I could hardly stand up. It was really hard, but it helped that my dad was there with me.

"Once I got home, I would get really tired. But I stayed in bed hardly at all. I was moving around the house, doing my walking exercises a lot. I didn't feel like doing my homework, but I had a homebound tutor who helped me. I also ate a lot. Because I'd lost about fifteen pounds after surgery, my mom fed me steak for breakfast, lunch, and dinner—which sounds good, but you do get sick of it after a while.

"Although the doctor said I could go back to school two weeks after surgery, I waited six weeks so I could start a new term. All the kids were really nice when I got back, and they hardly noticed my brace because it's so form-fitting. Even the really popular kids, the ones you don't think know who you are, said, 'Hey, Laney, we're glad you're back at school.' And the only class I had trouble catching up on was Spanish, but that's because everything you learn in a foreign language builds on everything else.

"The saddest thing to me is that I had to give up gymnastics. I never did think I was going to be all that great, but I just liked the sport. We went to meets three nights a week, out of town, and I miss seeing all those people. But now I'm taking up tennis—I've played three times since surgery—and I'm pretty good at it.

"Even though I was in a lot of pain after surgery—sometimes I thought I was going to die—I can hardly remember any of it now. My brace came off after only four months, I got an inch and a half taller, I've finally got a waistline, and now I'm straight. And in another couple of weeks, after the doctor has checked out my X rays, I'm looking forward to getting his permission to go water-skiing!"

Laney's mother, Catherine, looks forward to that day as well. For her, it will mark the end of the Moss family's bout with scoliosis, an experience that seemed to last "forever." Here, she shares some thoughts about what it's like to be the parent of a youngster who's going to have scoliosis surgery.

"We felt relieved when we learned that Laney could have surgery. We'd been living with the brace for such a long time, and it was uncomfortable, cumbersome, and hot for Laney. As a mother, it had hurt me to watch her wearing the Boston brace, and we'd had such problems trying to find her clothes that would fit—the brace made her waist three sizes bigger, but her hips were so tiny, everything would just fall to the floor. She accepted it pretty well— we had our 'Oscar designer clothes' and all—but it was hard for her. It seemed like she'd been in that brace forever, and we were glad that something else could be done for her.

"Her curve was just going wild. Over the summer, it increased 20 more degrees in her lower back, and she was getting a bad inward slope in the middle of her back. That scared me, because it increased even though she swam every day and was wearing a brace. I could tell how bad it was getting—when she'd dive in the swimming pool, her back would go crooked. And I knew if we didn't do something, it would only get worse.

"When we knew she was going to have surgery, we got on the ball right away to get things done, like having Laney donate her own blood for the surgery. But where we live, you can't donate blood if you're underage, so we had a lot of problems—it was almost as if it took an act of Congress. It can be done, though. We got permisison from our pediatrician and from the orthopedic surgeon, and had to go through the state Red Cross to get approval. Then we had to drive sixty miles every week to give the blood.

"My husband and I worked it out so that one of us was with Laney all the time she was in the hospital. I was able to stay near her overnight, and in the morning when I went back to the hotel to shower, my husband would come over and stay with her. I think it helped her a lot. When she had gas pains, I was there to rub her stomach and walk her up and down the halls with the I.V. still attached to her arm; and when she had to have the plaster mold put on, her daddy went with her. That seemed to make her feel better.

"Several things happened that made us all feel better. First, we brought our hometown orthopedic surgeon to the hospital so he could watch the surgery. We wanted to make sure he'd know what to do if we had problems once we got home. Second, everything was out in the open—everything that was told to my husband and me was told to Laney, and I think that's the way it should be. We never had any secrets, and I think that's why she handled it as well as she did. Third, our surgeon could bring himself down to the eye level of the patient. He commands respect, but he can communicate with a child. I liked that, and felt it was important to Laney.

"I know that some parents are afraid to bring their kids to the doctor. But the one thing I've learned through this is that you must take a child—or an adult, for that matter—to the doctor when she's healthy. That way you'll have records that you can refer to so you know what's wrong. If you wait until there's something wrong, it may be too late."

TWO SURGERIES STRAIGHTEN THE SPINE AND STRENGTHEN THE CHARACTER

Like many of the surgical patients I interviewed, I put off having surgery until I was an adult. I finally made the decision at the age of twenty, nearly five years after I had first sensed something was wrong with my back. That's unfortunate, because at the age of fifteen, my curve was probably only 20 degrees and could have been treated nonoperatively. By the time I met Dr. Bradford in 1970, my spine had twisted around to 43 degrees. I felt surgery was my only alternative.

My deformity was not obvious to the casual observer. I did not have the rib hump that's often associated with severe scoliosis, but my torso did seem to be twisting to the left, the result of a mild rotation of the vertebrae. And though my right shoulder was nearly an inch higher than the left, as was my hip, by deliberately leaning in the opposite direction, I could compensate for the asymmetry and make my body appear to be nearly level. Compensating for my crookedness, however, was a full-time, tiresome job; standing straight and level did not come naturally to me.

Curves like mine, in the 40- to 60-degree range, are not life-threatening. In most cases, they don't interfere with the heart or lungs and rarely do they cause pain. Indeed, many adults have curves of this magnitude, but they elect to do nothing about them. They can live with the fact that their bodies are slightly off-kilter. But there is a chance that curves can get worse during adulthood. That such a possibility existed was what made me decide to go ahead with surgery.

It was not an easy decision to make. I had just enrolled as a freshman at the University of Minnesota, and was working two part-time jobs as a legal secretary in order to finance my plans to one day become an English teacher. I'd also just met a fellow whom I thought would be the man of my dreams. Surgery threatened to ruin all of that. It would mean dropping out of school and work for a while (in those days, the standard recuperation period was at least a month), and since I'd have to wear a plaster body cast for nine months, I knew I'd be putting my newfound relationship in jeopardy. For weeks I was in agony: should I have the surgery and get "fixed," or should I gamble that my curve would stay right where it was?

On the strength of five years of painful memories and the sneaking suspicion that with my luck, the curve would worsen, I decided to go through with it. On the evening of January 15, 1970, I checked into Fairview-St. Mary's Hospital at five-feet-two, and by ten o'clock the next morning, thanks to Dr. Bradford's expert bone carpentry skills and the insertion of a Harrington rod, I was five-feet-four, though quite unconscious of my newly heightened stature.

When I finally awoke many hours later, one thought drifted through my mind: "I'm now two inches taller than I was a few hours ago." But as the anesthesia wore off and my body became more attuned to the realities of major surgery, all I could think of was pain. I felt as if someone were standing on my torso. I called for more pain medication and got it, then drifted back to sleep.

A few days later, when I started to feel a bit more alert, two nurses stood at my bedside and announced, "It's time for your log rolls." I didn't know what they were talking about, until one of them pulled up the sheet beneath me, and used it like a lever to roll me to the other side, where the other nurse stood ready to catch me.

"Don't do that!" I screamed. "I'm not ready to move yet! You're going to break my rod!" They assured me that log rolls were good for me. As for the Harrington rod hooked to my spine, they said it wouldn't break. "It's made of stainless steel," they said.

They were right. The rod didn't break, and by week's end, I came to look forward to seeing their cheery faces as they clutched at my sheet and shouted, "Alleee-ooop!"

I'd have gladly gone along with being rolled indefinitely if it had meant I could escape the next traumatic experience that awaited me. I was wheeled down to the cast room, where four orthopedic residents were preparing to slather my body with the sticky, smelly goop that would harden and become my body cast!

"What kind of body do you want?" they asked. "Voluptuous? Streamlined? If you've got the time, we've got the plaster." Jokesters, all of them. But their playful banter helped allay my fears as they removed my surgical gown, pulled a long body stocking over my head, and positioned it, like an elongated tube top, over two thirds of my shivering body. Unable to see what they were about to do—the top of the stocking covered my face to protect it from clouds of plaster dust—I prayed for time to pass quickly. Within minutes, they were patting and pulling long strips of plaster-soaked gauze around my neck and across my breasts, waist, and hips.

"More on the left!" one of them shouted. "Smooth down the buttocks," said another. "Aren't you finished yet?" I mumbled beneath my mask.

Twenty minutes later, the plaster had dried. I lay there on the table, my face finally exposed to the light, feeling like a mummy—cold, clammy, encased. But before I had a chance to whine about it, one of the residents was coming toward me with what looked like a little buzz saw.

"What are you going to do with that?" I gasped.

"Trim your hair, dummy," he said with a giggle. "Seriously, I'm just going to trim your cast. You want to look good in this, don't you?" He zipped off the excess plaster from around my neck, shoulders, and buttocks, then cut out a large oval from the plaster that surrounded my stomach.

"This will help you breathe easily," he said. "You'll be glad it's there after you eat. When your stomach expands, it'll have somewhere to go." When he finished with his nips and tucks, the group hoisted me back on the cart and returned me to my room.

I wasn't allowed to get out of bed yet, so I couldn't see what the cast looked like, but I was dying to know! Was it really as big as it felt? How was I going to conceal it? I was certain I looked hideous, but I wouldn't know for sure for another week.

"It's time to get out of bed and take your first walk," said my nurse about two weeks after the surgery. The news stunned me! I felt no more prepared to walk than I did to play football! But despite my protests, I soon found myself on the edge of the bed, my feet dangling toward the floor.

"Up you go!" said my nurse. "C'mon. You can do it!"

What a bizarre feeling to stand again! My knees were wobbling and I felt as if my body would buckle under the weight of the twelve-pound cast. Slowly I took one step, then another. Ten steps later, I was ready to sit down. But before I did, I managed to gather enough strength to walk to a mirror. I had to see what I looked like!

"Hideous!" I thought as I stroked the boxy mold that hid my otherwise tiny figure. "I look like a freak!"

No one could comfort me. Not the nurses, not Dr. Bradford, least of all my friends. They all said I looked fine ("for somebody who's just had spine surgery"), but I knew they were lying. I looked like a mummy, and sure as hell felt like one. I pleaded with Dr. Bradford to remove it, trying to convince him that I'd be really careful if I didn't have to wear one. But he was unfazed by my arguments. "It's there to protect you," he reminded me. "You never know what might happen."

I didn't think I'd be able to stand it. And it was going to be like this for the next nine months! I was angry, hurt, and depressed. But worse, I was worried. What would my new boyfriend do or say when he saw me like this?

I got my answer three weeks later when he came to pick me up for our first date since the surgery. We were going to a party at the home of one of his friends, people I'd never met. That made me nervous, but not as much as seeing my date. After all, he'd probably never seen a walking, talking mummy before!

To say that he looked surprised when he saw me would be an understatement. When I opened the door, he took one look at me and said, "Oh God, I didn't know it was going to look like that!" I tried to appear cheerful and even offered to let him sign my cast. "Maybe later," he said glumly as he led me to his car.

We rode in silence. His eyes were glued on the road, mine on the ceiling of the car. That was the only position I could sit in where the cast didn't pinch into my chin.

When we arrived at the party, I felt as if everyone was staring at me. Indeed, they probably were, since none of them had ever seen a person in a body cast.

"Doesn't it hurt?" "Aren't you hot?" "Do you really have to wear that thing for nine whole months?" Everyone had a question, and I got pretty sick of it if you want to know the truth. So after about half an hour of being grilled with queries, I fled to the bathroom and had a good cry. Finally I composed myself, yanked my turtleneck up over the neck piece one more time, and made my way down the basement stairs that led to the party room below.

Suddenly my ankle gave out on the second step and I fell back, sliding jerkily down the stairs on my back like a turtle skidding down a bumpy hill. The back of my head and my buttocks ached from hitting against the plaster as I made my descent. But nothing was hurt more than my pride.

They all flocked around me. "Are you all right?" "Are you hurt?" "Maybe somebody should call an ambulance!" Actually, that didn't strike me as such a bad idea—I wasn't seriously hurt, but I sure wanted to make a fast getaway!

My date wasn't much help. In fact, I think he was more embarrassed than I was. But at least he was quick on his feet; he had me in the car within minutes and we were on our way back to my apartment.

We didn't speak, aware that this was probably our last date. But the twenty-minute ride gave me time to come to two important, startling realizations. Any guy who couldn't see through plaster to find the person underneath just wasn't the guy for me. And now I knew that my ugly, cumbersome shell was there for a reason after all. It probably saved me from breaking my neck, my rod, or my back!

By the next week, I had returned to school and my jobs. No, it wasn't easy schlepping around campus with this heavy shell surrounding my body or craning my neck over the bulky mold in order to see what I was typing at work. I also disliked having to take sponge baths, and shampooing my hair meant getting into the bathtub on all fours with a plastic sheet wrapped around me to protect the plaster. The smell of sweaty plaster in the summer was enough to make me wretch; even dumping spoonfuls of Chanel No. 5 bathpowder down my back couldn't mask the odor! I hated the way I looked—I felt compelled to cover myself with turtlenecks and maternity tops, which only made me look worse, and pregnant. And sometimes I thought I'd go mad because of the itching. My solution to this problem was to stretch out a wire hanger, and try to slip it underneath my cast, but it usually ended up getting caught on the body stocking, whereupon I'd be forced to ask a neighbor to help me pull it out! But despite all these aggravations, time passed quickly, and before I knew it, I was back in Dr. Bradford's office. The day of the unveiling had finally arrived.

No sound has ever been lovelier to me than that of the small buzz saw he used to remove my cast. In minutes, it was split open and the dusty, frayed shell, now in halves, fell to the floor. Quickly I ran my hands along my back. It felt good. It felt straight. But would it bend?

Slowly I leaned over from the waist, my hands dangling toward the floor. No pain, just a little stiffness from being held imprisoned all those months. Next, with my hands on my hips, I twisted at the waist, then arched my back. No problem! By now, I couldn't even remember where Dr. Bradford had placed the rod along my spine. I knew only that I now had terrific posture! At that moment, it mattered little that a four-hour operation, a metal rod, and a plaster torture chamber had made it possible.

When I returned home that afternoon, I ripped off my turtleneck, vowed to burn it and every other piece of "cast clothing" I owned, and slid into a steamy bubble bath, where I giddily watched every square inch of my skin shrivel up like a prune. That first bath could well be entered in the *Guinness Book of World*

Records as the longest time any human has ever spent lounging in a tub! Then I spent several hours prancing nude around my living room, taking breaks every five minutes or so to admire my newly straightened body in the mirror. What a delightful time I had trying on all the clothes I hadn't worn for nearly a year and dreaming about all the new, slinky outfits I would buy that would adorn my lovely new body! To be sure, that day ranks among the top ten of my life!

Over the course of the next seven years, I finished my coursework at the university, completed my apprenticeship as a student teacher, and by 1977 was a full-fledged teacher of English at a high school in a suburb of Minneapolis. It was a year of triumph for me because it marked the first year of what I thought would be a lifetime career. But it was also a year of tragedy: the Harrington rod inside me broke, and once again I was faced with having to have surgery.

I firmly believe I know exactly when it happened, though Dr. Bradford contends that the rod probably began to wear out over a period of months, that it would be unlikely to suddenly snap, or that a person would actually feel it break. Both of us, however, agree on why it happened: a small portion of the bone graft had failed to fuse years before (in an area of my spine that was not easily seen on X ray), and this caused the rod to become dislodged and more susceptible to stress, the way a hairpin, if continually twisted, will eventually weaken and break.

One breezy summer evening, I was sitting in an overstuffed chair in my apartment, correcting huge piles of research papers I had assigned my students as their final project of the year. Suddenly I heard a crash in the next room and reeled around in my chair, certain that a burglar had climbed in through the bedroom window. Midway through my turn, I felt a hot pain shoot up my spine, not unlike the painful tingling sensation you feel when you turn your neck too quickly. Slightly dazed, I got up from my chair, tiptoed toward the bedroom, and saw that the wind had blown my tiny wind chime against the wall and shattered it. "Burglar, indeed," I thought. I began cleaning up the mess, but when I bent over to pick up the shards of glass, I felt that tingling sensation again.

When I awoke the next morning, my entire upper body felt stiff and my head throbbed. And in the days that followed, although the stiffness disappeared, the headache became my constant companion. Rest did not relieve the pain. Great quantities of aspirin had no effect. Nothing took the pain away.

Because it was my head, not my back, that hurt, it didn't occur to me at first that something might be wrong with my spine. In fact, when I finally made an appointment with a general practitioner, I never even mentioned that I'd had spine surgery. All I talked about was the throbbing in my head.

Believing that my problem was tension, the doctor wrote out a prescription for Valium, a muscle relaxant. Dutifully, I took one every four hours, but the drug didn't rid me of my headache; it only made me feel groggy and depressed.

After weeks of wooziness, I decided that my problem was not tension. God knows, popping all that Valium made my body feel like rubber most of the time! So I finally made an appointment with Dr. Bradford. Perhaps all this pain did have something to do with my back!

I'll never forget that day. Dr. Bradford sent me to the lab for X rays and when I returned to his office, I slipped on a flimsy paper gown while he quickly examined my body and listened to my tale of the twenty-four-hour-a-day headaches. My body checked out fine, he said, and so I stood behind a privacy screen and began getting dressed. In the meantime, a nurse delivered the X rays, and Dr. Bradford put them up on the light board. Just as I zipped up my slacks, I heard him say, "Hmmm, your rod's broken."

I peeked around the screen and looked at the X ray. Seemingly floating amid the cloudy-looking vertebrae was a rod—half of it secured in place against the spine, the other half jutting out at an angle where the break had occurred. "Surely that couldn't be *my* X ray," I thought. "That wasn't *my* rod, was it?"

Dr. Bradford gently assured me that the X ray and the rod indeed belonged to me.

"I'm sorry this happened," he said, pointing to the two pieces that were once a single shaft of metal. "It's happened because you've got a pseudarthrosis—one part of your fusion didn't take." I don't recall hearing him explain that when pseudarthrosis occurs, part of your spine buckles out and puts pressure on the rod, which in turn causes it to break. I only remember these words: "We're going to have to go back in and repair the fusion and put in a new rod."

(Note: Today, if an adult patient experiences pseudarthrosis or has another type of condition that requires a revision of a fusion, her surgeon may recommend that she wear a spinal stimulator after surgery for several hours a day for a period of three to five months. According to Dr. Frank Rand of Boston Children's Hospital, who notes that the electro-magnetic devices have been approved by FDA, "Although we're not quite sure why they work, spinal stimulators can improve a patient's fusion rate. We don't typically recommend its use for a first surgery, but if I were doing a revision of a fusion, or any type of fusion in the pelvic area, I'd definitely think about using it. Patients who think they might benefit from a stimulator should consult with their orthopedist.")

Quite frankly, I didn't care about the surgery or the rod. What mattered to me was the fact that, once again, I'd be enveloped in a plaster cast. Nine more months of looking like a cocoon!

I can't say I enjoyed this second ordeal, yet I have to admit I was pleasantly surprised at the way things turned out. In the seven years since I'd had my first surgery, doctors had changed their thinking about how postsurgical patients should be treated, so this time, instead of lying on my back in my body cast for weeks after surgery, I was up and walking after about three days. I was out of the hospital seven days later, and returned to teaching within two weeks, this time in a much thinner cast that just barely covered my collarbone and stopped at the middle of my hips.

Psychologically, I was a much stronger patient the second time around. During the seven months that I wore the cast, I didn't try to conceal myself in turtlenecks or maternity tops and, in fact, I made a conscious effort to dress just like anyone else, even if portions of the cast did peek through my clothes. I even got used to being teased by my students—they loved to tell me "knock-knock" jokes while rapping on my cast and shrieking, "Who's there?"

Of course, I wouldn't want to go through surgery again. Twice is enough for anybody! But what I gained from the experience of having two spine surgeries and wearing body casts for a total of sixteen months of my life has more than offset any of the fear, anguish, and pain I had to endure as the result of having had scoliosis. I'm not referring here to the physical benefits of surgery—the fact that I'm still two inches taller, have great posture, two evenly balanced shoulders, a clearly defined waist, and no longer have to struggle with clothes that don't seem to fit. What is important to me is the psychological and emotional strength I garnered along the way.

In ways that may be difficult for someone who hasn't had surgery to understand, scoliosis *can* strengthen your character. Who can fear a deadline or a test, a meeting or a confrontation, after one experiences and overcomes the fear of having a surgeon work so close to the spinal cord? Who can be plagued by self-consciousness in everyday situations after one has sported a brace—or a heavy plaster cast—all summer long? And who can be impatient with the little aggravations of daily existence after one has waited months to be released from a protective shell?

If you've never had great respect for the human body and your health, or taken your share of responsibility for these marvelous gifts of life, you're a lot like I was before I finally had to come to grips with the fact that I'd have to have surgery. But once you've taken steps to correct your scoliosis—by making an appointment with a specialist, being fitted for a brace, or going through with surgery if you need it—you'll be that much closer to taking control of your life, a long, happy, productive life that's the result of stopping scoliosis in time.

7

Searching for the Cause

Despite all the technological advances that have been made in the treatment of idiopathic scoliosis, its cause, or etiology, still eludes us. But that doesn't mean that orthopedic researchers haven't spent a good deal of time looking for clues.

For years they've peered into nearly every nook and cranny of the human body, trying to track down a logical reason why an otherwise perfectly healthy individual develops a spinal curvature. Yet for all their efforts, particularly those of the men and women who are members of the Scoliosis Research Society, the best explanation they've been able to come up with is that idiopathic scoliosis is probably a "multifactorial" disorder—in other words, there are many different elements that may contribute to the development of a scoliotic curve.

HEREDITY IS A FACTOR

Most of the evidence gathered so far seems to indicate that one factor can be found by studying genetics, the branch of biology that deals with heredity. According to Dr. Keim, idiopathic scoliosis "usually is transmitted by one or both parents to their offspring. Therefore, the child receives a 'dose' of scoliosis when the sperm and ovum combine. It's much like programming a computer to punch out a specific genetically coded message twelve or thirteen years later."

In Dr. Keim's orthopedic practice, for example, at least 60 percent of all the children he sees have a family history of scoliosis, and many children have brothers and sisters with the same condition. In fact, he says "in two families six siblings are involved, and in one family two children required surgery and three wear braces for scoliosis." In the course of my own research, I spoke with many youngsters and adults whose parents and siblings also had scoliosis, including one young woman from a family who had such a strong "dose" of scoliosis, not only did she and her parents have it, so did seven out of her eight brothers and sisters! In that family, two of the children had had surgery and two were recently fitted for Milwaukee braces.

If scientists are ever able to locate and identify the particular gene or genes that control the development of scoliosis, perhaps they'd be able to manipulate them via genetic engineering techniques and thus "deprogram" the body's genetic computer and prevent it from "printing out" the scoliotic message. Until that happens, they will continue to study other ways of getting at the causes.

Just how many possible causes are there? When I put that question to Dr. Alf Nachemson, professor of orthopedic surgery at the University of Goteborg in Sweden, who has surveyed the world literature on research into the causes, he scratched his head, smiled, took a very deep breath, and provided me with what he called a "mere sample" of causes that have been proposed over the years.

"Scoliosis patients have crooked mothers or crooked fathers, one leg is shorter than the other, or one arm is longer than the other. The scoliosis patients grow too quickly and menstruate too early, they cannot look straight with their eyes, and they do not talk intelligently. They have poor postural stability, their spinal nerves do not grow enough, and their muscles show asymmetrical strength."

Heaving a sigh, he continued. "Their muscles contain abnormal fibers, as well as viruslike bodies. Their body chemistry has gone haywire. Their vitamin C intake is too small, their sugar intake is too big. They have strange elastin fibers everywhere. Platelet abnormalities are also found in their blood. Their discs grow in the wrong direction, their spines become unstable, and their joints stiffen up."

Finally, as the lines of his face relaxed, he said, "I shall stop here, but I could actually continue for a long time."

Though I was fairly exhausted after scribbling down this fancy list of possible causes of idiopathic scoliosis, I was not surprised at its size. After all, why *should* there be only one causal explanation for a disorder that can present itself as a C- or S-shape in nearly a dozen curve patterns, some with more vertebral rotation than others? And how could just one cause explain why, for example, two nearly identical young ladies, both with a 30-degree curvature, will have completely different outcomes? One of them may go through life without her curve ever progressing another degree, while the other, even after wearing a brace for years, may eventually develop a curve of such magnitude that it can only be treated surgically.

NOT JUST ONE DISORDER

Such diversity has led many orthopedists and scientists to conclude that idiopathic scoliosis may not be just one disorder after all. Says Dr. Ogilvie: "Now we tend to lump most of these curves—C- and S-shaped, thoracolumbar patterns, and all the others, progressive and nonprogressive—into one category called 'idiopathic scoliosis.' But eventually, I think we're going to find that we're not dealing with the same disorder at all. In fact, I can't assure you that five to ten years from now we'll even be able to say that right and left curves are in the same category.

"This phenomenon has occurred in medicine before," he explains. "A hundred years ago, when researchers studied pneumonia, for example, they figured that whether people were coughing up blood or phlegm or fluid, they all had one disease called pneumonia. But now we know many different microbes can cause many different kinds of pneumonia and that they're really very different diseases. And by way of analogy, I think we'll find the same thing will be true of idiopathic scoliosis. But identifying the scoliotic disorders isn't going to be easy, because in many cases, when we discover some abnormality that presents itself in people with idiopathic scoliosis, we don't have the technology or the money to pursue it as far as we need to."

CLUES FROM THE BRAIN

Research into the etiology of scoliosis has unearthed a variety of abnormalities within people who have the disorder. For example, researchers at the University of Rochester School of Medicine have found differences in the right and left hemispheres of the brain in people who have idiopathic scoliosis.

In most people, the left side of the brain controls language and mathematical ability, whereas the right side processes information necessary to perform musical and artistic activities. To find out which side of a person's brain is dominant for language, scientists will place earphones on a subject through which the person hears a series of phonetic syllables. Then the person is asked to record the sounds she hears through either ear. "We consider these sounds to be elements of language," explains Dr. Kurt Enslein, former director of the Center for Research in Scoliosis at the University of Rochester, "and so we ask subjects to write down the sounds they hear to reveal which half of the brain is dominant for language. When the left half is dominant, more of the sounds they write down have been presented to the right ear; when the right half is dominant, more are presented to the left."

So far, Dr. Enslein and his colleagues have tested approximately seventy youngsters with idiopathic scoliosis in just this way and have found that "they're not likely to be left dominant for language, but rather bilateral or right dominant." Dr. Enslein says that when similar tests were performed on youngsters without scoliosis, the individuals had left dominance for language. Although many more studies will have to be conducted in this area, Dr. Enslein believes that if this theory can be proven, "Eventually, this fifteen-minute listening test could provide us with an early indicator of kids at risk of developing scoliosis."

If you're wondering why researchers would look for a cause in such a seemingly unlikely place as the brain, it's because a lot of the research that has focused on more obvious places—such as the tissues surrounding the spine, and the vertebral discs—has not yet produced the "right" answer.

COLLAGEN ABNORMALITIES

For example, scientists have done a great deal of research on *collagen,* a substance that is found in nearly all body tissues, including muscle, bone, tendons, vertebral discs, and skin, and that literally holds our bodies together. They've performed this research because they know that in certain rare diseases, such as *Marfan's syndrome* and *Ehlers-Danlos syndrome,* a collagen defect that weakens the tissues surrounding the spine can cause scoliosis. As you might have guessed, they have found abnormalities in the collagen of people with idiopathic scoliosis, but their most current studies indicate that the curvature probably causes the abnormality in collagen, not vice versa.

At the University of Minnesota, Dr. Bradford and his colleague Dr. Theodore Oegema, a professor of orthopedic surgery and biochemistry, have looked at other connective tissues that contain collagen—the discs that are wedged between the vertebrae of the spine.

According to Dr. Oegema, the first symptom of scoliosis is that the interior of the discs shifts to one side and the discs become wedge-shaped. When the doctors began their research, they hypothesized that this wedging eventually forced the spine to curve, and so they looked for reasons why the disc would shift in the first place.

This meant they had to look deep within the discs at *proteoglycans,* molecules that act like sponges to soak up nearby water molecules. When the proteoglycans collect a proper amount of water, they plump up evenly like cushions and prevent the vertebrae from grinding together. If they collect too little water, they can shrink and flatten; and if they soak up an overabundance of water, they can balloon on one side or the other. Perhaps, the doctors reasoned, proteoglycans were at the root of scoliosis. If they could just find a way to change the ability of these molecules to attract water, they'd be able to even out the discs and the vertebrae that surround them.

In the last several years, Drs. Bradford and Oegema and other researchers have learned that changes in the discs of people with scoliosis probably occur as a result of biomechanical changes in the spine—not because the discs are somehow inherently abnormal or diseased. Despite this radical change in their thinking, they still believe that if misshapen discs could be altered, they could either stop a curve from progressing or straighten it to some extent. Toward that end, the researchers have been experimenting with an enzyme that may be able to correct misshapen discs. Called *chymopapain*—a substance purified from papaya plants—it interferes with the water-holding ability of proteoglycans. By injecting the enzyme into the discs of laboratory animals, they've found that they partially can change the shape of the discs. Says Dr. Oegema: "If we can understand the nature of this process, it may be possible to enhance it and develop a treatment for scoliosis that will give a more normal back as an end result. This would involve identifying at an early stage patients who will not respond to the usual treatments. These patients would be treated in an as yet undefined manner to optimize disc recovery. This would allow reconstitution of the disc in a normal manner and function. These goals are long-term, but exciting."

Indeed, the prospect of being treated with an enzyme—perhaps by being given an occasional injection of chymopapain—would be a welcome alternative to youngsters whose only nonsurgical treatment option at present is to wear a brace until they reach skeletal maturity. But imagine how delighted they'd be if researchers could prove that scoliosis is caused by a dietary deficiency—perhaps then their only involvement in "treatment" would be gulping a few extra vitamin or mineral supplements each day!

DIET MAY PLAY A ROLE

That notion may seem farfetched, but researchers at the University of California at Davis have performed studies in which diet modification appears to influence the severity and progression of scoliosis in susceptible animals. Studies involving dietary copper led them to publish a paper in the July 1984 issue of *Science,* in which they concluded that "the identification of copper as an environmental factor with the potential of influencing the expression of scoliosis is important. At the very least, our observations suggest that diet plays a role in the etiology of idiopathic scoliosis."

The scientists, including Drs. Robert Rucker, Ursula Abbott, Christina Kenney, and William Upsahl, came to their conclusions after studying the effects of dietary copper on a genetic strain of White Leghorn chickens that develop scoliosis. Many of the features of scoliosis that occur in this animal correspond to those observed in humans. For example, the Leghorns' curves often occur in the thoracic area of the spine, and they appear to develop before the animal is sexually mature—the avian equivalent to the adolescent growth spurt. Says Dr. Rucker, "It is important to emphasize that the birds studied are genetically susceptible to expressing scoliosis . . . and that manipulating their diet appears to *change* that susceptibility." Recent work by Rucker's group indicates that in addition to copper, deficiencies of manganese and vitamin B-6 also worsened the birds' scoliosis.

According to Dr. Rucker, the theory behind the group's interest in copper evolved from a basic understanding of—you guessed it— collagen. "A large majority of protein in bone is made up of collagen fibers that are cross-linked (held together chemically). This process is initiated by an enzyme called lysyloxidase," he explains. "We know that with poor cross-link formation, the bone weakens. Since copper is part of the cross-linking enzyme, we thought if there was a defect in copper metabolism, then perhaps this could lead to a defect in the vertebrae which would allow a curvature to develop."

When they reduced the level of copper fed to the animals each day, the researchers found that they not only could produce scoliosis (of at least 10 degrees) in 90 percent of the Leghorns after twelve weeks, they could also manipulate the severity of the curves—some Leghorns that received the least amount of copper developed curves of 40 to 50 degrees.

While the Californians' findings suggest a link between diet and scoliosis, let's not forget that the experiments were performed on chickens, not humans. Also, these genetically susceptible chickens develop mild scoliosis *whether or not* there is dietary manipulation. As such, the study may have little to say about the effects of diet on people who have or may develop idiopathic scoliosis. Dr.

Rucker puts it into perspective: "I'm not willing to say that in humans, scoliosis is a problem because a given nutrient intake is deficient. To take data from chickens and apply it to humans is not easily done. But our work does introduce the possibility that diet in some susceptible individuals may be one part of the etiological puzzle of scoliosis."

Even though vast amounts of etiological research have been conducted on animals, scientists are often leery of the conclusions that are suggested by them. Says Dr. Ogilvie: "You can take Japanese quail or certain strains of salmon or Leghorn chickens and deprive them of copper or other things and you can create scoliosis. But the question is: what relationship does experimental scoliosis have to idiopathic scoliosis? Experiments have been performed on rabbits that caused scoliosis in them, but what does that mean? A rabbit has a horizontal spine and a man has a vertical spine, so what happens in an experiment with a rabbit may or may not have an application to humans. To be sure, animal research is vitally important, but it's not applied research. The best theories now available about the etiology of scoliosis come from studies done on 'bipedal ambulators'—in other words, human beings."

ABNORMAL BACK MUSCLES

One of those theories is that idiopathic scoliosis is a muscle disorder. Many investigators have studied the back muscles that control spine position in both normal people and those with scoliosis. Some have studied such muscles by recording their electrical activity, while others have examined their biochemistry or microscopic structure. In most cases, researchers have found there are abnormalities that are present in the back muscles of people with idiopathic scoliosis.

In fact, when researchers biopsy the paraspinal muscles of scoliotic patients, they often find an abnormal ratio of *fast-twitch* and *slow-twitch fibers*—the fibers in humans that correspond to those in the light and dark meat of turkey. Dr. Ogilvie says: "The varying response rates of these muscles causes an imbalance—one side becomes strong, while the other side becomes weak—hence, a curvature forms."

Although most scientists now agree that people with idiopathic scoliosis have muscle problems, a crucial question still remains unanswered, namely, are these muscle problems the reason the curve develops, or do they occur because of the curve?

It may be that the nerves that control the muscles are the real culprits. Or perhaps the villain is the brain—it is, after all, the organ that orchestrates the way in which our muscles hold our bodies upright and in balance. That may sound like a far-reaching notion, yet several researchers today are trying to prove the notion that the brain and the spinal cord—together termed the *central nervous system*—are at the root of the cause of idiopathic scoliosis.

Before we explore this fascinating possibility, let's take a look at how the nervous system is organized and how it controls body posture and muscular movements.

UNDERSTANDING THE NERVOUS SYSTEM

Like a computer that is constantly being fed data, your brain—the prime mover behind your ability to stand up straight, keep your balance, and coordinate your bodily movements—constantly receives an enormous stream of information from sensory nerves throughout the body. Consider the sensory nerves involved with vision, for example. Let's say you're going to walk a straight line from one end of your living room to the other. As you do so—assuming you keep your eyes open during your travels—your optic nerves transmit messages to the brain about your body's motion and position and help keep you on a level course. But if you blindfolded your eyes, thus depriving your optic nerves (and your brain) of vital sensory information, and tried again to saunter along that imaginary straight line, you'd veer off your course and probably stumble into chairs, walls, or people!

Although there's no question that our sense of sight is at the forefront of conscious awareness, it is not the only source of information necessary to keeping us in balance and in control of our body position. If it were, then people who are blind would not be able to walk and maintain normal posture, nor would sighted people, when blindfolded, be able to sit and stand properly and perform any number of complex motor activities such as dribbling a basketball, playing the piano, or skipping rope. In fact, there are a variety of sensory systems other than vision that provide our brains with important information that allows for the maintenance of balance and posture.

If you've ever spun around in circles and then stopped quickly, you've no doubt experienced a feeling of great dizziness, and of disorientation with your surroundings. The sensory system that creates these sensations is located deep within your ear in an area called the "inner ear." It is usually referred to as the *vestibular apparatus,* or balance mechanism, and it consists of several thin fluid-filled canals and sacs that are lined with tiny hairs which arise from nerve cells called *neurons.*

Each time you move your head and change its position, the fluid in the canals shifts and causes those tiny hairs to bend. When this happens, the neurons fire off electrical signals to the brain which provide it with information about the angle of your head and how the rest of your body is positioned in relation to it. With this information, your brain then stimulates the muscles of your body to react in such a way that you continue to stand upright. In fact, if your brain did not receive this vestibular information, it's likely that every time you leaned your head to one side, you'd have trouble keeping your balance.

It's important to note that your vestibular and visual systems often work together to provide balance and proper posture. When your brain receives messages from the neurons in the inner ear, it can instruct your eyes to change their position in relation to the objects in your visual field while your body is in motion. Thanks to this working partnership, you're able to keep a fixed gaze on your friend while you move toward her.

As you walk toward your friend, other complex and crucial sensory systems are hard at work sending messages to your brain. One of these is called the *proprioceptive system,* a network of sensors located in the ligaments and other soft tissues of all your joints. Whether you're moving or standing still, these sensors send information to the brain about what your joints are doing at any particular moment and where they're positioned in relation to the rest of your body.

Other sensors within the body provide *tactile* data, or information about touch. For example, such sensors within the skin of your feet send messages to your brain that tell it whether you're standing on a surface that is flat, inclined, stationary, or moving.

You'd think the circuitry of the brain would be overloaded by the time it had processed all this complex data. Not so! In fact, the brain has the ability to pack even more information into its data bank from yet another elaborate group of sensors—the body's motor-control system that sends and receives messages related to the degree of stretch and tension each muscle in the body is experiencing.

When you're reaching for an apple, for instance, your brain sends a message to the muscles of your arm that says, in effect, "Muscles, you must reach six inches in order to get to that apple." Your muscles receive this message and begin to extend themselves; then they send back a message to the brain that says, "Is this far enough?" Your brain now uses this information to fine-tune the reach until the hand finally grasps the apple.

Although this motor-control sensory information is not a part of the apparatus that is concerned with detecting body position, the information it provides is crucial to the brain's ability to direct the muscle activity responsible for holding the body upright and in balance.

All of the information transmitted by these various sensory systems is received, processed, and integrated by the central nervous system in phenomenal quantities with incredible speed. While you walk down the street, engrossed in a pleasant daydream, the central nervous system is working at a fever pitch to maintain posture, balance, and smooth walking.

But what does all this have to do with scoliosis? There is growing evidence that an abnormality in the nervous system, related to the control of posture, may be the causal factor in some, or perhaps all, persons with idiopathic scoliosis.

It is well known that a variety of neurologic conditions and diseases such as cerebral palsy and polio can cause scoliosis. They do this, presumably, by disrupting the delicate balance of the muscles that keep the spine straight under normal circumstances. Once a sufficient muscular imbalance occurs, the forces on the spine are skewed, and a curvature results. And if this occurs at a time when the spine is growing, normal patterns of growth will be disrupted and a permanent scoliosis can result.

Researchers probing along these lines have shown that they can produce scoliosis in animals whose nervous systems have been somehow damaged. While this knowledge has furthered our understanding of how nervous system or neurologic diseases can cause the spine to curve, it does not answer the critical question: is there some specific neurological abnormality that is the cause of, or contributes to, idiopathic scoliosis? The answer is probably years away, but researchers around the world are hard at work in their laboratories right now trying to find it.

REFLEX MECHANISMS MAY BE THE CULPRIT

Many of the medical professionals involved with studies of the central nervous system theorize that idiopathic scoliosis is caused by a primary neurological disturbance, and they are focusing their attention on the reflex mechanisms that maintain posture and are involved with all the sensory information sent to the brain by the visual, vestibular, tactile, proprioceptive, and motor-control systems.

Although much of the work in this area was pioneered by Dr. Kengo Yamada and his colleagues in the department of orthopedic surgery at Tokushima University in Japan, some of the most recent research has been conducted here in the United States by Dr. Richard Herman, who is now the medical and research director at Good Samaritan Regional Medical Center in Phoenix, Arizona.

Based on numerous experiments, Dr. Herman believes that people with idiopathic scoliosis suffer from a disturbance in "visual-spatial perception." In other words, despite the fact that all the body's sensory systems are sending messages to the brain, it does not interpret correctly how upright the body is. Thus, even though sensory data may be saying, in effect, "This human body is standing straight from top to bottom and is in a correct position relative to its environment," the brain scrambles the message. Now it is faced with a conflict between visual information and the data received from the inner ear and the sensors on the joints. But the brain doesn't sit idly by and accept all this confusion; instead, it tries to reduce the conflict by reinterpreting the sensory information. The net result is that the brain interprets a straight spine as being curved, and while it believes it is coordinating muscle activities to keep the spine vertical, in actuality it is causing the spine to curve. So while the brain is able to compensate for a disturbance in visual-spatial perception, it does so at the cost of producing scoliosis.

It may seem downright bizarre, if not impossible, that the brain can reorganize information in this way. Yet researchers—or your high school science teacher—could prove to you that it does, in fact, occur. If you were to put on a pair of prism glasses, you would quickly discover that everything in your visual field—the floor, a table, the ceiling—appears tilted. But within a short period of time, you would "adapt" to this new environment by unconsciously tilting your head to correspond with the tilted surroundings. Your brain, however, would convince you that your head was in a normal, vertical position! According to Dr. Herman and his colleagues, it is just this sort of unconscious phenomenon that occurs when a person has idiopathic scoliosis, although the "environment" that the brain of a scoliotic person responds to is not a room that seems tilted, but a spine that seems curved.

In order to gain more evidence about the neurologic abnormalities that may cause scoliosis, Dr. Herman has studied patients' ability to maintain their balance when they're standing still, or when some sort of movement occurs beneath them. To do this, he places individuals on a *stabilometer,* a plate that can be made to move in a regular and predictable motion, or in a random or sudden fashion. Attached to the plate are sensors that can detect how often and how much a subject shifts her balance or moves her feet when the plate is set in motion.

By placing patients on the stabilometer in various ways and recording information from the sensors, Dr. Herman can get a pretty good idea of how much each sensory system contributes to a person's overall postural control and equilibrium. For example, he will blindfold his subjects so that their brains can no longer rely upon visual information; in these instances, the *tactile sensors* of the feet and *proprioceptive sensors* of various muscle groups become the primary messengers to the brain. On other occasions, he will give the vestibular apparatus the most rigorous workout by moving the plates in an unpredictable fashion.

From these sorts of experiments, Dr. Herman has found that when the stabilometer remains at rest, scoliotics seem to demonstrate better balance than normal children. But when there's movement involved, scoliotic children in general lose their balance more easily than non-scoliotic youngsters. In fact, the greatest loss of balance occurs when the stabilometer moves unpredictably—a time when a person's visual-vestibular systems should be working in high gear to try to prevent bodily imbalance. To Herman and his colleagues, this finding suggests that the visual-vestibular system is not functioning as it should. They believe this malfunctioning reflects a brain disturbance that ultimately causes the curve to develop.

In order to add more evidence to his theory that the central nervous system is at the root of scoliosis, Dr. Herman has also studied what is known as the *vestibulo-ocular reflex (VOR)*, the rapid to-and-fro eye movements that occur when a person tries to keep her eyes on an object while moving her head in a circular motion. Remember, as the eyes dart back and forth, visual information is being sent to the brain, and as the head moves in different directions, the fluid in the inner ear shifts, causing those neurons to fire off their messages as well. In these experiments, Dr. Herman found the VOR abnormal in youngsters with scoliosis and, in fact, those subjects with the most severe curves had the most abnormal VOR.

Taken all together, these findings have led Dr. Herman and his colleagues to conclude that idiopathic scoliosis is due to a primary defect in the central nervous system. Yet there are a number of orthopedic surgeons and scoliosis researchers who take issue with this theory on the grounds that one exasperating question still remains unanswered: is the defect in the central nervous system actually causing the curve, or is the curve causing a defect in the central nervous system? Perhaps, they reason, these central nervous system abnormalities are the result of a normal brain trying to adapt to an abnormal situation.

In a recent interview with Dr. Herman, I learned that he is closer than ever to unraveling the truth about the cause of idiopathic scoliosis. In fact, having just concluded a six-year study, he now says he has sufficient evidence to corroborate his initial theory, i.e., that idiopathic scoliosis is caused by a defect in the central nervous system. Perhaps most important, he claims that roughly 75 percent of the time, his tests can accurately predict who will get scoliosis and who will not.

Dr. Herman's study, which was funded by the National Institutes of Health, involved roughly 120 youngsters who were on average nine years of age. "If we had attempted a study within the general population," he explains, "where roughly one person in a thousand is likely to get idiopathic scoliosis, we'd have had to find an enormous number of subjects in order to get a sufficient statistical number. Therefore, we selected a group of adolescents who were siblings (brothers or sisters) of individuals who had scoliosis. This meant that all the youngsters in our study had a high risk of developing scoliosis. Of course, at the beginning of the study, six years ago, all these youngsters had straight spines."

To make his study as accurate and unbiased as possible, Dr. Herman chose what's called a "double-blind" design—in other words, he and his staff did not examine the children prior to testing, nor did they receive any information from the kids' parents or doctors. "We simply tested the youngsters," he says, noting that he used many of the techniques discussed earlier in this chapter.

After the tests were completed and the results tabulated, Dr. Herman and his colleagues set about to make their predictions: who in the group would develop a curve, and who would not? Then they waited for nature to take its course—a period of about four years. "From the youngsters' doctors," he says, "we eventually received clinical reports which indicated who had actually developed a curvature and who had not. Then we compared these outcomes with our initial predictions. Not only did we score pretty well, but our predictions were also specific and selective: 75 percent of the time, we accurately predicted who developed scoliosis and who didn't."

As you might have guessed, Dr. Herman's study also revealed that those individuals who developed scoliosis had "a marked abnormality" in areas such as processing of visual and vestibular information. "These and other abnormalities were revealed *prior* to the development of curvatures," he notes, "which strongly suggests that a dysfunction in the central nervous system is involved in the development of idiopathic scoliosis."

Exactly which part of the brain is responsible? Dr. Herman isn't certain, but he is now beginning another study that may help him pinpoint the culprit. When and if he finds the precise area of the brain that causes a curve, he says, "I think we can design low-cost equipment for orthopedists and nurses to use to define the probability of a child developing a curve."

If that happens, what would preventive treatments be like? "In the ideal," says Dr. Ogilvie, "there would be a much more elegant treatment than bracing or surgery. It would be some sort of neurological treatment, a brain stem retraining device—almost like alpha waves—that would allow us to control the righting reflex that keeps a person balanced. We could use this device on people who are beginning to show signs of scoliosis, and perhaps we could even use it long before a curve ever appeared, as part of a program of scoliosis prevention for very young children. Perhaps we could use it to predict who will get scoliosis."

Even though research into the etiology of idiopathic scoliosis is vitally important because it could one day deliver the cure that thousands of people have been waiting for, there is another type of research that, for the moment, has a greater impact on you and your life than any that is being performed in a laboratory at a medical school. It is the personal research that you're willing to do concerning your own body. And that means watching for the signs of scoliosis—the tilted shoulder, the uneven hemline, the hint of a hump along the back—then immediately seeing a doctor to get a professional examination. If you do that for yourself or for a loved one, you'll be taking an active role in what is the common goal of all lay people, orthopedists, and researchers: stopping scoliosis!

Appendix A:
Recommended Reading

Resources from the National Scoliosis Foundation

The following is a list of resources that the National Scoliosis Foundation (NSF) recommends for parents and young people. Orders should be sent to the National Scoliosis Foundation, 72 Mt. Auburn St., Watertown, MA 02172.

The Brace and *Her Brace Is No Handicap.* An illustrated short story and a true story, each concerns a teenage girl coping successfully with scoliosis. *The Brace* was written by Mary Langford; *Her Brace Is No Handicap* was written by Carolyn Callison. Both are reprints from *Young Miss* magazine. Write to NSF and include $1.00 for a single copy.

Getting a Second Opinion. A reprint from *Health Tips*, a publication of the California Medical Education and Research Foundation. For a single copy, send a self-addressed, stamped (25-cent stamp), business-size envelope.

NSF General Packet. Packet contains general information on scoliosis. Write to NSF for details.

NSF Adult Packet. Packet contains information of interest to adults with scoliosis. Write to NSF for details.

1 in Every 10 Persons Has Scoliosis. This brochure explains what scoliosis is and how to screen for it. It also contains facts about the

Foundation. For a single copy, send a self-addressed, stamped (25-cent stamp), business-size envelope. Specify English or Spanish version when writing to NSF.

Reprints of *Medical Update* column from *The Spinal Connection.* Reprints are available on the following topics: Adult Scoliosis; Scoliosis and Pregnancy; Answers to Questions about Mild Curves: Electrical Stimulation; Cotrel-Dubousset Technique; X rays; Understanding Medical Terminology. Send a self-addressed, stamped (25-cent stamp), envelope to NSF and specify topic of interest.

Scoliosis . . . Now it can be treated in adults as well as children. A reprint from *Cleveland Magazine.* For a single copy, send a self-addressed, stamped (25-cent stamp), business-size envelope to NSF.

A Scoliosis Patient Becomes a Model. A reprint from *Children's Today,* a publication of The Children's Hospital, Boston. For a single copy send a self-addressed, stamped (25-cent stamp), business-size envelope.

The Spinal Connection. A newsletter published by the National Scoliosis Foundation that is published in the spring and fall. It is full of interesting articles concerning the Foundation, plus a *Medical Update* column that discusses facts about scoliosis. Contact NSF for subscription information.

Straightened Back, Strengthened Character. Written by Paul Dienhart, it is a reprint from the Summer 1983 issue of *Health Sciences,* a publication of the University of Minnesota. For a single copy, send a self-addressed, stamped (25-cent stamp), business-size envelope.

The Treatment of Spinal Curvature. Written by Kathleen Doheny, it is an in-depth article for the layman concerning current treatment for abnormal spinal curvature. First printed in January 1987. Send a self-addressed, stamped (25-cent stamp), business-size envelope along with $1.00 to NSF.

Additional Resources

The following pamphlets may also be helpful. Note that all orders must be prepaid in United States currency and mailed to the addresses listed below.

Adult Scoliosis Surgery . . . It Can Be Done. A booklet describing various types of surgery for the adult scoliosis patient. Covers the two-stage spine fusion, halo-traction, and other techniques. $4.50 for a single copy. Order from St. Luke's Spine Center, 11311 Shaker Boulevard, Cleveland, OH 44104.

Adult Spinal Deformity. A basic handbook for adult patients that discusses scoliosis and kyphosis. Send $.50 to the Scoliosis Research Society, P.O. Box 2001, Park Ridge, IL 60068.

The AMA Book of Back Care. A book of information on back care compiled in 1982 by the American Medical Association. Cost is $12.95. Write Random House, 201 East 50th Street, New York, NY 10022.

Backtalk. A newsletter for parents and young people. Write the Scoliosis Association, Inc., P.O. Box 51353, Raleigh, NC 27609 for information on subscription rates.

Brace Yourself. Third edition, $3.00 each (100 or more, $2.50 each). Write St. Luke's Spine Center, 11311 Shaker Boulevard, Cleveland, OH 44104.

Going Home. Instructions for pediatric and adult patients who have had a spinal fusion. Includes fourteen inserts to choose from in order to meet the patient's individual needs. $2.50 each. Write the University Hospital Spine Center, 2074 Abington Road, Cleveland, OH 44106 for a list of inserts.

Reducing Patient Exposure During Scoliosis Radiology. Available cost-free from the Food and Drug Administration. Write FDA/HFZ, Rockville, MD 20857 and ask for Order Number FDA 85-8252.

Scoliosis. A brochure describing the cause, prevention, and treatment of scoliosis, kyphosis, and lordosis. Write for details concerning cost to the American Academy of Orthopaedic Surgeons, P.O. Box 618, Park Ridge, IL 60068.

Scoliosis—A Handbook for Patients. Offers information on the detection and treatment of adolescent and adult scoliosis, kyphosis, and lordosis. $1.50 each. Write the Scoliosis Research Society, P.O. Box 2001, Park Ridge, IL 60068.

Scoliosis and Kyphosis. Provides information and advice for the parents of scoliosis patients. $.50 each. Write the Scoliosis Research Society, P.O. Box 2001, Park Ridge, IL 60068.

Scoliosis! Me? An illustrated pamphlet by Dr. Richard A. Marks that gives detailed answers to questions most asked by parents. Cost is $2.50

each. Write to the North Dallas Scoliosis Center, 1910 North Collins Boulevard, Richardson, TX 75080.

Scoliosis Road Map. Written for teenagers, the pamphlet unfolds to a 22-inch by 23-inch poster. $1.50 each. Write the University Hospital Spine Center, 2074 Abington Road, Cleveland, OH 44106.

Scoliosis Surgery: What's It All About? The pamphlet answers many of the questions patients ask before having surgery. $.75 each. Write the University Hospital Spine Center, 2074 Abington Road, Cleveland, OH 44106.

What If You Need an Operation for Scoliosis? Third edition, $3.00 each (100 or more, $2.50 each). Write St. Luke's Spine Center, 11311 Shaker Boulevard, Cleveland, OH 44104.

What Young People and Their Parents Need to Know About Scoliosis. Information from a physical therapist's perspective. $1.00 for a single copy. (50 copies for $34.50 requires prepayment and a $2.00 shipping and handling cost.) Write the American Physical Therapy Association, 1111 No. Fairfax St., Alexandria, VA 22314.

When the Spine Curves. Available cost-free from the Food and Drug Administration. Write FDA/HFZ, Rockville, MD 20857 and ask for Order Number FDA 85-4198.

You and Your Brace. $.75 each. Write the University Hospital Spine Center, 2074 Abington Road, Cleveland, OH 44106.

Appendix B:
Scoliosis Organizations

NATIONAL SCOLIOSIS FOUNDATION, INC.
72 Mt. Auburn St.
Watertown, MA 02172
(617) 489-0880
President: Laura B. Gowen

Founded in 1976, the National Scoliosis Foundation (NSF) is a nonprofit organization devoted to alerting the public to the potentially serious health problems associated with abnormal spinal curvatures, and to promoting early detection and timely preventive professional treatment through the screening of every child aged ten to fifteen, the critical growth years.

To reach its goal of eliminating the effects of abnormal progressive spinal curvatures, the staff and volunteers of NSF maintain a resource center; work in close cooperation with writers, publishers, and producers; make presentations to appropriate groups; and provide easy-to-read literature for individuals, health centers, schools, and spine clinics. In addition, they are consultants for persons interested in required school screenings and have testified before legislative committees when invited. NSF also publishes a biannual newsletter, *The Spinal Connection,* and provides information on guidelines and materials for implementing and improving screening programs with follow-up for parents. The Foundation has produced an educational unit on scoliosis for the prescreening education of students in fifth through seventh grades. This includes an audiovisual presentation, teacher's guide, poster, brochure, and resource sheets listing sources for additional materials. For more information, write to NSF at the above address.

THE SCOLIOSIS ASSOCIATION, INC.
P.O. Box 51353
Raleigh, NC 27609
(919) 846-2639
President: Barbara M. Shulman

Founded in 1976 by the parents of scoliosis patients, the Scoliosis Association is a nonprofit organization. It has among its goals educating the general public about scoliosis and other spinal deviations. It also encourages and sponsors scoliosis screening programs. To obtain information on the publications, films, and tapes available, write to the association directly.

The Scoliosis Association publishes a newsletter, *Backtalk,* four times a year. All members of the chapters and the association receive this newsletter, which prints news likely to be of interest to scoliosis patients and others in medical and educational fields. For information about membership applications and dues, write to the association.

The association also sponsors the formation of scoliosis chapters throughout the country. These chapters are parent/patient support groups that afford the scoliosis patient and his or her family a meeting place every month with other families involved with scoliosis. At these meetings, members can help one another to effect a positive social and emotional adjustment during the treatment of scoliosis. To find out if there is a support group in your area, call or write the headquarters of the Scoliosis Association at the above address.

SCOLIOSIS RESEARCH SOCIETY
Suite 127
222 South Prospect Avenue
Park Ridge, IL 60068
(708) 698-1627

Founded in 1966, the Scoliosis Research Society (SRS) is a non-profit organization composed of orthopedic surgeons and spine specialists who are dedicated to education, research, and treatment of spinal deformities. The SRS also sponsors an annual meeting that is a forum for the presentation of the most current research results. The organization is an affiliate of the American Academy of Orthopaedic Surgeons, and it publishes a number of informative materials on scoliosis. For more information about available publications and films, write to the SRS.

AMERICAN ACADEMY OF ORTHOPAEDIC SURGEONS
222 South Prospect Avenue
Park Ridge, IL 60068
(708) 823-7186

The American Academy of Orthopaedic Surgeons (AAOS) is a not-for-profit organization founded in 1933. AAOS is the largest medical organization for musculoskeletal specialists. Members of the academy have completed medical school and up to five years of specialty study in orthopedics in an accredited residency program, passed a comprehensive oral and written exam, and have been certified by the American Board of Orthopaedic Surgery.

AAOS is committed to increasing the public's awareness of musculoskeletal conditions such as scoliosis, with an emphasis on preventive measures. For more information about available AAOS publications, contact the Communications and Publications Department there.

Appendix C:
Where to Get Help

This section lists hospitals, medical centers, clinics, and doctors who treat patients with scoliosis. Although great care was taken to include as many names as possible, it should be noted that this list is by no means complete. Entries followed by an asterisk (*) indicate that the doctor's office is situated in a location other than a hospital or clinic and you must inquire as to the particular hospital or clinic affiliation.

All doctors and institutions included on the list responded to a written survey. Nevertheless, it is wise to contact the various offices directly for information on services available. Unless otherwise indicated, doctors and institutions treat both children and adults.

This information—which is not intended as an endorsement of any individual or institution—is meant to be a starting point for patients and their families. You may wish to seek a second or third opinion.

Alabama

Flowers Hospital
P.O. Box 6907
Dothan 36302

Orthopedic Clinic, P.A.
P.O. Box 5949
Dothan 36302

Southeast Alabama Medical
  Center
P.O. Box 6987
Dothan 36302

The Center for Orthopaedic
  Specialties, P.A.
3715 Dauphin St.
Mobile 36608

Arizona

Associated Orthopedic Surgeons
5402 East Grant Rd., B1
Tucson 85712

Children's Rehabilitative Services
124 West Thomas Rd.
Phoenix 85013

Howard H. Ginsburg, M.D.*
222 West Thomas Rd., Suite 307
Phoenix 85013

Good Samaritan Medical Center
  and Phoenix Children's
  Hospital
1111 East McDowell Rd.
Phoenix 85006
(Treats patients up to age 19)

Humana Hospital
1947 East Thomas
Phoenix 85016

Terry E. McLean, M.D.*
3330 North Second St., Suite 102
Phoenix 85012

Phoenix Spine Center
1331 North Seventh St.
P.O. Box 13648
Phoenix 85002
(Treats patients up to age 19)

San Raphael Orthopaedics
6506 East Carondelet Dr.
Tucson 85710

St. Joseph's Hospital and Medical
  Center
350 West Thomas Rd.
Phoenix 85013

The Orthopedic Clinic
2700 North Third St., Suite 100
Phoenix 84004

Tucson Medical Center
5400 East Grant Rd.
Tucson 85712

Tucson Orthopaedic & Fracture
  Surgery
1779 West St. Mary's Rd.
Tucson 85745

Arkansas

Arkansas Back Clinic, P.A.
9600 Lile Dr., Suite 280
Little Rock 72205

Arkansas Children's Hospital
800 Marshall St.
Little Rock 72202
(Treats patients from 1 to 21)

Arkansas Spine Center
5 St. Vincent Circle, Suite 305
Little Rock 72205

Baptist Medical Center
9601 Interstate 630, Exit 7
Little Rock 72205

California

Behrooz Akbarnia, M.D.*
8010 Frost, Suite 401
San Diego 92123

Daniel R. Benson, M.D.*
2230 Stockton Blvd.
Sacramento 95817

John Carlisle Brown, M.D.*
361 Hospital Rd., Suite 523
Newport Beach 92663

Cedars Sinai Medical Center
8637 West Third St., Room 940E
Los Angeles 90048

Central Coast Spine Institute
862 Meinecke
San Luis Obispo 93405

Children's Hospital and Health
  Center
8001 Frost St.
San Diego 92123
(Treats patients up to age 18)

Children's Hospital, Los Angeles
Scoliosis Clinic
4650 Sunset Blvd.
Los Angeles 90027
(Treats children and young
  adults)

Children's Hospital of Orange
  County
455 South Main St. North
Orange 92668

Children's Hospital of San
  Francisco
P.O. Box 3805
San Francisco 94119

Eureka Orthopaedic Medical
  Group, Inc.
2826 Harris St.
Eureka 95501

Steven S. Fountain, M.D.*
360 Dardanelli Lane, Suite 1F
Los Gatos 95030

Fountain Valley Regional
  Hospital
Orthopaedic Medical Clinic, Inc.
11100 Warner Ave., Suite 368
Fountain Valley 92708

Gallatin Medical Clinic
10720 South Paramount Blvd.
Downey 90241

John M. Gray, M.D.*
3838 California St., Room 111
San Francisco 94118

Hoag Hospital
301 Hospital Rd.
Newport Beach 92663

John Muir Medical Center
1601 Ygnacio Valley Rd.
Walnut Creek 94598

Kaiser Hospital–Oakland
280 West MacArthur Blvd.
Oakland 94611

Kaiser Permanente Medical
  Center
280 West MacArthur Blvd.
Oakland 94611

Thomas A. Kuh, Jr., M.D.*
360 Dardanelli Lane, Suite 1F
Los Gatos 95030

Thomas T. Laughlin, Jr., M.D.*
9900 Genesee Ave., Suite C
La Jolla 92037
(Treats patients from age 1 to 80)

Raymond Jay Linovitz, M.D.*
9900 Genesee Ave., Suite C
La Jolla 92037

Norman Livermore, M.D.*
120 La Casa Via
Walnut Creek 94598

Loma Linda University Spinal
   Deformities Clinic
Loma Linda University Medical
   Center
11234 Anderson Street
Loma Linda 92350

William C. McMaster, M.D.*
1310 Stewart, Room 508
Orange 92668

Orthopaedic Hospital Scoliosis
   Clinic
2400 South Flower St.
Los Angeles 90007

Orthopaedic Specialists
2001 Santa Monica Blvd., Suite
   360W
Santa Monica 90404

Pacific Spine Clinic, Inc.
355 East Grand Ave.
Escondido 92025

Palomar Medical Center
Escondido 92025

Pediatric Orthopaedics Assoc.
800 South Fairmont Ave., Suite
   300
Pasadena 91107
(Treats patients up to age 20)

Pleasanton Orthopaedics
5565 West Las Positas, Suite 320
Pleasanton 94566

Presbyterian Intercommunity
   Hospital
12401 East Washington Blvd.
Whittier 90602

Robert Rovner, M.D.*
5601 Norris Canyon Rd., Suite
   101
San Ramon 94583

San Dieguito Orthopaedic
   Medical Group, Inc.
Spinal Surgery Associates
1087 Devonshire Dr., Suite 311
Encinitas 92024
                -or-
9900 Genesee Ave., Suite C
La Jolla 92037

Scripps Memorial Hospital
9888 Genesee Ave.
La Jolla 92037

Scoliosis Center of San Diego
8008 Frost St., Room 208
San Diego 92123
(Treats patients up to age 25)

Scoliosis Clinic
Children's Hospital
747 Fifty-Second St.
Oakland 94609
(Treats patients up to age 18)

Shriners Hospital
1701 Nineteenth Ave.
San Francisco 94122
(Treats patients up to age 21)

Sierra Vista Hospital
1010 Murray
San Luis Obispo 93405

Peter Slabaugh, M.D.*
3300 Webster, Room 1200
Oakland 94609

Southern California Complex
Spine and Scoliosis Center
12401 East Washington Blvd.
Whittier 90602

Spinal Deformity Clinic
Rancho Los Amigos Medical
  Center
7601 East Imperial Highway
Downey 90242

St. John's Hospital
2428 Santa Monica Blvd., Room
  201
Santa Monica 90404

St. Joseph Hospital
Delbeer St.
Eureka 95501

St. Luke Medical Center
2632 East Washington Blvd.
Pasadena 91107

David E. Taylor, M.D.*
6107 North Fresno St., Room
  102
Fresno 93710

Robert G. Treat, M.D.*
400 Newport Center Dr., Room
  506
Newport Beach 92660

University of California, Davis
School of Medicine
Department of Orthopaedics
2317 Stockton Blvd.
Sacramento 95817

University of California,
Los Angeles Scoliosis Clinic
10833 Le Conte Ave.
Los Angeles 90024

University of California, San
  Francisco,
Department of Orthopedic
  Surgery
533 Parnassus Ave., U-471
San Francisco 94143

Valley Children's Hospital
3151 North Millbrook Ave.
Fresno 93703

Valley Presbyterian Hospital
Scoliosis Center
15107 Van Owen St.
Van Nuys 91409

Colorado

Children's Orthopaedics South
6979 South Holly Circle, Suite
  275
Englewood 80112
(Treats patients up to age 21)

Fitzsimons Army Medical
  Center
Department of Pediatrics
Adolescent Clinic
Aurora 80045
(Treats patients up to age 21)

Bertram Goldberg, M.D.*
601 East Hampden, Suite 180
Englewood 80110

Lakewood Orthopaedic Clinic,
  P.C.
1805 Kipling St.
Lakewood 80215

Orthopedic Associates
801 North Cascade Ave.
Colorado Springs 80903

Orthopaedic Center of the
    Rockies
2500 East Prospect
Fort Collins 20525

Penrose Hospital
Cascade Ave.
Colorado Springs 80903

Poudre Valley Hospital
1024 Lemay Ave.
Fort Collins 20525

St. Anthony Hospital Center
1805 Kipling St.
Lakewood 80215

The Children's Hospital
1056 East Nineteenth Ave.
Denver 80218
(Treats patients up to age 21)

Woodridge Orthopaedic Clinic
3550 Lutheran Parkway West
Wheatridge 80033

Connecticut

Michael J. Murphy, M.D.*
60 Temple St.
New Haven 06510

Newington Children's Hospital
181 East Cedar St.
Newington 06111

Yale New Haven Hospital
New Haven 06510

Delaware

Alfred I. duPont Institute
Department of Orthopaedics
1600 Rockland Rd.
Wilmington 19899
(Treats patients up to age 21)

Ali Kalamchi, M.D.*
1941 Limestone Rd., Suite 209
Wilmington 19808

District of Columbia

Children's Hospital, George
    Washington Hospital, and
    Washington Hospital Center
901 Twenty-Third St., N.W.
Washington 20037

Children's National Medical
    Center
Department of Orthopaedics
111 Michigan Ave., N.W.
Washington 20010
(Treats patients to age 18)

Peter A. Moskovitz, M.D.*
3 Washington Circle, N.W.,
    Room 404
Washington 30027

Orthopaedic Surgery Service
Walter Reed Army Medical
    Center
6825 George Avenue, N.W.
Washington 20307

Florida

Arnold Palmer Hospital for
    Children and Women
92 West Miller St.
Orlando 32806

Baptist Medical Center
4237 Salisbury Rd.
Jacksonville 32216

Bayfront Medical Center
(All Children's Hospital)
701 Sixth St. South
St. Petersburg 33701-9985

Florida Elks Children's Hospital
P.O. Box 49
Umatilla 32784
(Treats patients up to age 16)

Florida Hospital
601 East Rollins St.
Orlando 32803

Florida Orthopaedic Institute
4175 East Fowler Ave.
Tampa 33617

Flynn Orthopaedic Clinic
100 West Gore St., Suite 403
Orlando 32806

Hobby, Rowley, Smith and
Davis, P.A.,
615 Eleventh St. North
St. Petersburg 33705

Jewett Orthopedic Clinic
1285 Orange Ave.
Winton Park 32789

Matthews Orthopaedic Clinic
1315 South Orange Ave., Second
floor
Orlando 32806

Miami Children's Hospital
3200 Southwest 60 Ct., Suite 105
Miami 33155

Mount Sinai Medical Center
4300 Alton Rd.
Miami Beach 33140
(Treats patients from 1 to 18)

Nemours Children's Clinic
P. O. Box 5720
Jacksonville 32247
(Treats patients up to age 21)

Orlando Regional Medical
Center
1414 South Kuhl Ave.
Orlando 32806

Orthopaedic Rehabilitation
Associates
4237 Salisbury Rd., Suite 203
Jacksonville 32216

Shriners Hospital for Crippled
Children
12502 North Pine Dr.
Tampa 33612
(Treats patients to age 21)

University of Miami/Jackson
Memorial Medical Center
Box 016960
Miami 33155

Georgia

Children's Orthopaedics of
Atlanta
5455 Meridian Mark Rd., Suite
440
Atlanta 30342
(Treats patients up to age 21)

Emory Clinic
1365 Clifton Rd., N.E.
Atlanta 30322

Grady Memorial Hospital
80 Butler St., S.E.
Atlanta 30303

Peachtree Orthopaedic Clinic
2001 Peachtree Rd., N.E.
Atlanta 30309

Savannah Scoliosis Clinic
7 St. Joseph's Professional Plaza
Savannah 31419

Scottish Rite Children's Medical
  Center
1001 Johnson Ferry Rd.
Atlanta 30342
(Treats patients up to age 21)

St. Joseph's Hospital
11706 Mercy Blvd.
Savannah 31419

University Hospital
820 St. Sebastian Way
Augusta 30910

Hawaii

Shriners Hospitals for Crippled
  Children
Scoliosis Clinic
1310 Punahou St.
Honolulu 96826
(Treats patients from birth to 21)

Straub Clinic & Hospital
888 South King St.
Honolulu 96813

Illinois

Carle Clinic
602 West University Ave.
Urbana 61801

Carle Foundation Hospital
611 West Park
Urbana 61801

Charles F. Eberle, M.D.*
301 North Eighth St.
Springfield 62701

Loyola University of Chicago
2160 South First Ave.
Maywood 60153

Lutheran General Hospital
1775 Dempster St.
Park Ridge 60068

Memorial Medical Center
Department of Surgery
P.O. Box 19230
Springfield 62794

Methodist Medical Center of
  Peoria
221 Northeast Glen Oak Ave.
Peoria 61636

Michael Reese Hospital
Thirty-First St. at Lake Shore
  Dr.
Chicago 60616

Northwestern Memorial
  Hospital
Department of Orthopaedics
211 East Superior Ave.
Chicago 60611

Orthopaedics and Scoliosis, Ltd.
1725 West Harrison, Suite 472
Chicago 60612

Parkside Orthopaedics
1875 Dempster St.
Park Ridge 60068

Pediatric Orthopedic Surgery
  Center
18811 Dixie Hwy.
Homewood 60430
(Treats patients up to age 21)

Pediatric Orthopaedics and Spine
  Surgery
1 South 224 Summit, Suite 207
Oakbrook Terrace 60181
(Treats patients up to age 35)

Rush Presbyterian St. Luke's
  Medical Center
1653 West Congress Pkwy.
Chicago 60612

Charles M. Slack, M.D.*
30 North Michigan Ave., Suite
  1718
Chicago 60602
       -or-
7126 North Lincoln Ave.
Lincolnwood 60646

Spine Clinic, Shriners Hospital
  for Crippled Children
2211 North Oak Park Ave.
Chicago 60635
(Treats patients up to age 21)

St. Francis Hospital, Evanston
355 North Ridge
Evanston 60202

The Spine Center, Ltd.
614 North Sixth St.
Springfield 62702

Wyler Children's Hospital
General Pediatric Clinic
5841 South Maryland Ave.
Chicago 60637
(Treats patients up to age 18)

Indiana

James Whitcomb Riley Hospital
  for Children
702 Barnhill Dr.
Indianapolis 46202

Methodist Hospital of Indiana
1701 North Senate Blvd.
Indianapolis 46202

N.E. Orthopaedics, Inc.
5050 North Clinton
Fort Wayne 46825

Orthopaedic Surgery Group
1633 North Capitol Ave., Suite
  536
Indianapolis 46202

Orthopaedics Indianapolis, Inc.
Methodist Hospital
1801 North Senate Blvd., Suite
  200
Indianapolis 46202

Parkview Memorial Hospital
2200 Randallia Dr.
Fort Wayne 46825

Pediatric Orthopedic Surgery
  Center
1650 Forty-Fifth St.
Munster 46321
(Treats patients up to age 21)

George F. Rapp, M.D.*
8402 Harcourt Rd., Room 809
Indianapolis 46260

Riley Children's Hospital
702 Barnhill Dr.
Indianapolis 46202
(Treats patients up to age 16)

St. Francis Hospital
The Spine Institute
1500 Albany, Suite 705
Beech Grove 46107

St. Mary's Medical Center
3700 Washington Ave.
Evansville 47750

St. Vincent Hospital
2001 West 86th St.
Indianapolis 46260

St. Vincent Carmel Hospital
13450 North Meridian St., Suite
   275
Carmel 46032

Tri-State Orthopaedic Surgeons,
   Inc.
801 St. Mary's Drive, Suite 110
Evansville 47715

Iowa

University of Iowa Hospital
Department of Orthopedics
Carver Pavillion (First Floor)
Iowa City 52242

Kansas

Pediatric Orthopaedic Surgery
   Assoc.
5520 West College Blvd.
Overland Park 66211
(Treats patients up to age 21)

Orthopaedic & Reconstructive
   Surgery, P.A.
905 North Emporia
Wichita 67214

University of Kansas Medical
   Center
Thirty-Ninth Ave. and Rainbow
   Blvd.
Kansas City 66103

Wesley Medical Center
550 North Hillside
Wichita 67208

Wichita Clinic
3311 East Murdock
Wichita 67208

Kentucky

Kosair Childrens Hospital
231 East Chestnut St.
Louisville 40202

Leatherman Spine Clinic of The
   Norton Hospital
200 East Chestnut St.
Louisville 40202

Norton Hospital
601 South Floyd St., Room 200
Louisville 40202-1874

Shriners Hospital for Crippled
   Children
1900 Richmond Rd.
Lexington 40502
(Treats patients up to age 18)

University of Kentucky Medical
   Center
800 Rose St.
Lexington 40536

University of Kentucky Medical
   Plaza
E101, Division of Orthopaedic
   Surgery
Lexington 40536

Louisiana

Children's Hospital
200 Henry Clay Ave.
New Orleans 70118

Fox-Dean-Smith Orthopedics
873 Jordan St.
Shreveport 71101

Orthopaedic Clinic of Monroe
312 Grammont St.
Monroe 71201

Schumpert Medical Center
915 Margaret Pl.
Shreveport 71101

Shriner's Hospital for Crippled
    Children Scoliosis Clinic
3100 Samford Ave.
Shreveport 71103
(Treats patients up to age 18)

St. Francis Medical Center
309 Jackson St.
Monroe 71210-1901

Tulane Medical Center
1415 Tulane
New Orleans 70112

Maine

Rogers C. Southall, M.D., P.A.*
15 Lowell St.
Portland 04102

Mario Turi, M.D.*
404 State St.
Bangor 04401

Robert B. Keller, M.D.*
Cobb Medical Building
Belfast 04915
(No surgical treatment)

Maryland

Annie Arundel Orthopaedic
    Surgeons
Annie Arundel Medical Center
25 Shaw St.
Annapolis 21401

Children's Hospital and Center
    for Reconstructive Surgery
Scoliosis Clinic
3901 Green Spring Ave.
Baltimore 21211

James Lawrence Kernan Hospital
The Spinal Deformities Clinic
2200 North Forest Park Ave.
Baltimore 21207

Johns Hopkins Hospital
Scoliosis Clinic
600 North Wolfe
Baltimore 21205

Prince George's Orthopaedics
9440 Pennsylvania Ave.
Upper Marlboro 20772

St. Joseph's Hospital
    Orthopedic Associates, P.A.
1217 St. Paul St.
Baltimore 21202

University of Maryland Hospital
22 South Greene St.
Baltimore 21207

Massachusetts

Beth Israel Hospital
330 Brookline Ave.
Boston 02215
(Treats patients age 15 and above)

Children's Hospital
Spinal Deformities Clinic
300 Longwood Ave.
Boston 02193
(Treats patients up to age 21)

Lakeville Hospital
Main St.
Lakeville 02347

Massachusetts General Hospital
Pediatric Orthopaedic Unit
ACC 507
Boston 02114

New England Baptist Hospital
125 Parker Hill Ave.
Boston 02120

New England Medical Center
750 Washington St.
Boston 02111

Newton Wellesley Hospital
2014 Washington St.
Newton 02162

Woh H. Oh, M.D.*
One Brookline Place, Suite 503
Brookline 02146

Salem Hospital
81 Highland Ave.
Salem 01970
(Treats patients up to age 18)

Salem Orthopedic Surgeons
9 Colby St.
Salem 01970
(Treats patients up to age 18)

Shriner's Hospital for Crippled
    Children
516 Carew St.
Springfield 01104
(Treats patients up to age 18)

Alexander M. Wright, M.D.*
830 Boylston St.
Chestnut Hill 02167

Seymour Zimbler, M.D.*
993 Watertown St.
W. Newton 02165

Michigan

Borgess Medical Center
1717 Shaffer Rd., Suite 124
Kalamazoo 49001

Maurice E. Castle, M.D.*
6001 West Outer Drive, Suite 121
Detroit 48235

Childrens' Hospital of Michigan
3901 Beaubien Blvd.
Detroit 48201
(Treats patients up to age 18)

Grittenton Hospital
1000 West University Dr., Suite
    207
Rochester 48063

Henry Ford Hospital
Department of Orthopaedic
    Surgery
2799 West Grand Blvd.
Detroit 48202

Mary Free Bed Scoliosis Clinic
235 Wealthy St., S.E.
Grand Rapids 49503

Mt. Carmel Hospital
6071 West Outer Drive
Detroit 48235

Scoliosis Clinic
1521 Gull Rd.
Kalamazoo 49001

University Hospital
Section of Orthopaedic Surgery
TC-2914/0328
Ann Arbor 48109-0328

Wm. Beaumont Hospital
3023 North Woodward Ave.
Royal Oak 48072

Wm. Beaumont Hospital
   Scoliosis Clinic
3601 West Thirteen Mile Rd.
Royal Oak 48072

Minnesota

Abbott Northwestern Hospital
800 East 28th St.
Minneapolis 55407

Gillette Children's Hospital
200 East University Ave.
St. Paul 55101

Hennepin-Metropolitan Medical
   Center
701 Park Ave.
Minneapolis 55415

Mayo Clinic
Department of Orthopedic
   Surgery
200 First St., S.W.
Rochester 55905

Metropolitan Orthopaedic
   Associates
825 South Eighth St.
Minneapolis 55404

Minnesota Spine Center
606 Twenty-Fourth Ave. So.
Minneapolis 55454

Orthopaedic Consultants, P.A.
7373 France Ave. So., Suite 312
Edina 55435
(Treats patients up to age 20)

Riverside Medical Center
2312 South Sixth St.
Minneapolis 55454

St. Mary's Hospital
1216 Second St., S.W.
Rochester 55902

Twin Cities Scoliosis Spine
   Center
2737 Chicago Ave. So.
Minneapolis 55407

University of Minnesota
   Hospital
420 Delaware St., S.E.
Minneapolis 55455

Mississippi

Mississippi Spine Clinic
c/o St. Dominic Hospital
971 Lakeland Dr.
Jackson 39216

Pediatric Orthopaedic
   Specialists of Mississippi, P.A.
Suite 204 Medical Arts East
1190 North State St.
Jackson 39202-2413

University Medical Center
2500 North State St.
Jackson 39216-4505

University Orthopaedic
  Associates
University Medical Pavilion
1410 East Woodrow Wilson Dr.
Jackson 39216-5197

Missouri

Barnes Hospital
1 Barnes Hospital Plaza, Suite
  11300
St. Louis 63128

Children's Hospital
400 South Kings Hwy.
St. Louis 63110
(Treats patients up to age 18)

Children's Mercy Hospital
2401 Gillham Rd., Suite 2162
Kansas City 64108-9898
(Treats patients up to age 21)

Jewish Hospital
216 South Kings Hwy.
St. Louis 63178

Kansas City Orthopedic Clinic,
  Inc.
6724 Troost
Kansas City 64131

North Kansas City Hospital
2800 Hospital Dr.
No. Kansas City 64116

Parkway Orthopedic Group
456 North New Ballas
St. Louis 63141

Spine & Scoliosis Surgery, Inc.
2750 Hospital Dr.
North Kansas City 64116

St. Anthony's Hospital
10010 Kennerly Rd.
St. Louis 63128

St. Louis County Orthopedic
  Group
12615 Old Tesson Rd.
St. Louis 63128

University of Missouri Hospital
1 Hospital Dr.
Columbia 65212

Montana

Missoula Orthopedic Associates
700 West Kent
Missoula 59801

St. Patrick's Hospital
500 West Broadway
Missoula 59801

Nebraska

Immanuel Medical Center
6901 North Seventy-Second St.
Omaha 68122

Orthopedic Surgery Inc.
9110 West Dodge Rd.
Omaha 68114

Orthopaedic Surgery, Inc.
290 Embassy Plaza
Omaha 68114

University of Nebraska Medical
  Center
427 West Dodge Medical
  Building
8300 Dodge St.
Omaha 68114
                    -or-
Dept. of Orthopaedic Surgery
600 South Forty-Second St.
Omaha 68198-1080

New Hampshire

Davis W. Clark, M.D.*
280 Pleasant St.
Concord 03301

Concord Hospital
250 Pleasant St.
Concord 03301

New Jersey

Robert Fernand, M.D., P.A.*
516 Hamburg Tpk.
Wayne 07470

William A. Matarese, M.D.*
516 Hamburg Tpk.
Wayne 07470

Monmouth Medical Center
    Scoliosis Clinic
300 Second Ave.
Long Branch 07740
(Treats patients up to age 18)

Nadel Scoliosis Clinic
New Jersey Orthopaedic
    Hospital
289 Central Ave.
Orange 07050

Orthopaedic Surgery Assoc.
519 South Orange Ave.
South Orange 07079

New Mexico

New Mexico Orthopaedic
    Associates
415 Cedar, S.E.
Albuquerque 87106

Presbyterian Hospital
1100 Central Ave., S.E.
Albuquerque 87106

New York

Albany Medical College
Division of Orthopaedic Surgery
Albany 12208

Albany Memorial Hospital
Northern Blvd.
Albany 12203

Buffalo General Hospital
100 High St.
Buffalo 14203

Children's Hospital of Buffalo
Spine Clinic
219 Bryant St.
Buffalo 14222
(Treats patients up to age 21)

Columbia Presbyterian Medical
    Center
161 Fort Washington Ave.
New York 10032

East Huntington Orthopedic
    Group—Scoliosis Clinic
166 East Main St.
Huntington 11743

Gordon L. Engler, M.D.*
530 First Ave.
New York 10016

P. William Haake, M.D.*
220 Alexander St., Room 100
Rochester 14607

Stanley Hoppenfeld, M.D.*
1180 Morris Park Ave.
Bronx 10461

Hospital for Special Surgery
  Scoliosis Clinic
535 East Seventieth St.
New York 10021

Huntington Hospital
Park Ave.
Huntington 11743

Jack D. Weiler Hospital of the
  Albert Einstein College of
  Medicine
1825 Eastchester Rd.
Bronx 10461

Kings County Hospital Scoliosis
  Clinic
451 Clarkson Ave.
Brooklyn 11203

Maimonides Medical Center
4801 Tenth Ave.
Brooklyn 11235

Alan Moskowitz, M.D.*
784 Washington Ave.
Albany 12203

Mount Sinai Medical Center
5 East Ninety-Eighth St.
New York 10029

Jeffrey Muhlrad, M.D.*
1174 Route 112
Port Jefferson Station 11776

Nassau County Medical Center
  Scoliosis Clinic
Hempstead Tpke.
East Meadow 11756

Michael G. Neuwirth, M.D.*
1095 Park Ave.
New York 10028

New York University Medical
  Center
530 First Ave.
New York 10021

North Shore Orthopaedic &
  Spine Associates
1025 Northern Blvd.
Roslyn 11576

North Shore University Hospital
300 Community Dr.
Manhasset 11030

Orthopaedic Institute, Hospital
  for Joint Disease
211 East Seventieth St.
New York 10021

Our Lady of Mercy Medical
  Center
600 East 233rd St.
Bronx 10466

Scoliosis Clinic,
  Hospital for Joint Disease
301 East Seventeenth St.
New York 10021

St. Charles Hospital
200 Belle Terre Rd.
Port Jefferson 11777

State University of New York
Health Science Center at
  Brooklyn
450 Clarkson Ave.
Brooklyn 11203

State University of New York
Health Science Center at
  Syracuse
550 Harrison Center, Suite 100
Syracuse 13202

The Bronx Lebanon Medical
    Center Scoliosis Clinic
1650 Selwyn Ave.
Bronx 10457

The Genesee Hospital
224 Alexander St.
Rochester 14607

University of Rochester, Strong
    Memorial Hospital
601 Elmwood Ave.
Rochester 14642

Leonard S. Weiss, M.D.*
2920 Hempstead Tpke.
Levittown 11756

Richard L. Weiss, M.D.*
191 North St., Suite 110
Buffalo 14201

Westchester County Medical
    Center
19 Bradhurst Ave.
Hawthorne 10532

Martin Wolpin, M.D.*
2470 East 16th St.
Brooklyn 11235

North Carolina

Asheville Orthopedic Assoc.
111 Victoria Rd.
Asheville 28801

Bowman Gray School of
    Medicine
300 South Hawthorne Rd.
Winston-Salem 27103

Duke University Medical Center
Lenox Baker Children's Hospital
3000 Erwin Rd.
Durham 27705

Durham-Chapel Hill
    Orthopaedic Clinic
1828 Hillandale Rd.
Durham 27704

Gaul Orthopedic Group
2600 East Seventh St.
Charlotte 28204

Miller Orthopaedic Clinic—
    Scoliosis Center
1001 Blythe Blvd.
Charlotte 28103

North Carolina Spine Center
    P.A.
101 Conner Dr., Suite 200
Chapel Hill 27514

Orthopaedic Hospital of
    Charlotte
1901 Randolph Rd.
Charlotte 28207

Surgical Private Diagnostic Clinic
Duke South, Trent Dr.
Duke University Medical Center
Durham 27710

North Dakota

Dakota Hospital & Clinic
1702 South University Drive
Fargo 58102

Ohio

Akron City Hospital
525 East Market St.
Akron 44309

Children's Hospital of Akron
281 Locust St.
Akron 44308

Children's Hospital
One Children's Plaza
Dayton 45404

Children's Hospital
700 Children's Dr.
Columbus 43205

Children's Hospital Medical
    Center Spinal Deformity
    Center
Elland and Bethesda Aves.
Cincinnati 45229
(Treats patients up to age 18)

Cincinnati Orthopaedic Institute
2415 Auburn Ave.
Cincinnati 45219

Cleveland Clinic Foundation
9500 Euclid Ave.
Cleveland 44195

Elyria Memorial Hospital
630 East River St.
Elyria 44035
(Treats patients up to age 50)

John R. Kean, M.D.*
255 Taylor Station Rd.
Columbus 43213

James T. Lehner, M.D.*
5300 Far Hills Ave., Suite 100
Dayton 45429

Metro Health Medical Center
3395 Scranton Rd.
Cleveland 44109
(Treats patients up to age 18)

Northwest Ohio Spinal
    Deformity Center
St. Vincent Medical Center
2213 Cherry St.
Toledo 43608
(Treats patients up to age 21)

Outpatient North Clinic
9560 Children's Dr.
Mason 45040
(Treats patients up to age 18)

Rainbow Babies and Children's
    Hospital
2074 Abington Rd.
Cleveland 44106
(Treats patients up to age 18)

St. Luke's Hospital Spine Center
11311 Shaker Blvd.
Cleveland 44104

University Hospital of Cleveland
    Scoliosis Clinic
2074 Abington Rd.
Cleveland 44106

Reinhard A. Westphal, M.D.*
931 Chatham Lane
Columbus 43221

Oklahoma

Children's Hospital of Oklahoma
940 Northeast 13th St.
Oklahoma City 73126

Oregon

Bay Orthopaedic & Fracture
   Clinic, P.C.
2330 Broadway
North Bend 97459

Portland Orthopedic Clinic
3025 North Vancouver Ave.
Portland 97227

Sacred Heart Hospital
1200 Hilyard St.
Eugene 97401

Donald J. Schroeder, M.D.,
   P.C.*
1180 Patterson St.
Eugene 97401

Pennsylvania

Children's Hospital of Pittsburgh
3705 Fifth Ave.
Pittsburgh 15213
(Treats patients up to age 18)

Harrisburg Hospital
3916 Trindle Rd.
Camp Hill 17011

Jefferson Orthopaedic Associates
111 South Eleventh St., 8001
   New Hospital
Philadelphia 19107
(Treats patients up to age 21)

David P. Kraus, M.D.*
1350 Locust St., Suite 300
Pittsburgh 15219

Oakland Orthopedic Assoc.
5820 Centre Ave.
Pittsburgh 15206

Pennsylvania Hospital
800 Spruce St.
Philadelphia 19107

Scoliosis Clinic, University
   Hospital
Hershey Medical Center
Hershey 17033

Shriners Hospital
8400 Roosevelt Blvd.
Philadelphia 19152
(Treats patients up to age 21)

Temple University Hospital
Department of Orthopedics
3401 North Broad St.
Philadelphia 19140

Thomas Jefferson University
   Hospital
1015 Walnut St., 501 Curtis
   Clinic
Philadelphia 19107
(Treats patients up to age 21)

University of Pennsylvania
   Scoliosis Center
Thirty-Fourth and Civic Center
   Blvd.
Philadelphia 19104

Puerto Rico

John M. Flynn, M.D., F.A.C.S.*
Cobian Plaza Building GM-12
1607 Ponce de Leon Ave.
San Juan
(Treats children up to age 21)

Rhode Island

Rhode Island Hospital
593 Eddy St.
Providence 02903

South Carolina

Greenville Memorial Hospital
701 Grove Rd.
Greenville 29605

Piedmont Orthopaedic Clinic
1050 Grove Rd.
Greenville 29605

Tennessee

Baptist Memorial Hospital
899 Madison Ave.
Memphis 38146

Hugh P. Brown, M.D.*
979 East Third St., Room 805
Chattanooga 37403

Campbell Clinic, Inc.
869 Madison Ave.
Memphis 38103-3433

Erlanger Medical Center
979 East Third St.
Chattanooga 37403

Knoxville Orthopaedic Clinic,
    P.A.
1128 Weisgarber Rd.
Knoxville 37909

Suburban Orthopaedics, P.C.
3051 Lebanon Rd., Suite 111
Nashville 37214

Vanderbilt Orthopaedics Clinic
Vanderbilt University Medical
    Center
Nashville 37232

Texas

Ambulatory Care Center
Children's Hospital, Santa Rosa
    Medical Center
519 West Houston
San Antonio 78207

Austin Orthopedic Clinic
c/o Breckenridge Hospital
3100 Red River
Austin 78705

Baylor University Medical
    Center
3500 Gaston
Dallas 75246

Cook/Ft. Worth Children's
    Medical Center
801 Seventh Ave.
Ft. Worth 76104

El Paso Orthopaedic Surgery
    and Sports Medicine Group
1700 Murchison
El Paso 79902

Fort Worth Bone and Joint Clinic
1651 West Rosedale, Suite 100
Fort Worth 76104

Houston Northwest Medical
    Center
710 Form Marketing Rd. 1960
Houston 77090

Humana Advanced Surgical
    Institute
7777 Forest Lane, Suite C-707
Dallas 75230

Methodist Hospital
Orthopedic Department
6560 Fannin (2090)
Houston 77030

North Dallas Scoliosis Center
1910 North Collins Blvd.
Richardson 75080
(Treats patients age 10 and above)

Richardson Medical Center
401 West Campbell Road
Richardson 75080
(Treats patients age 10 and above)

Santa Rosa Medical Center
414 Navarro
San Antonio 78205

Jay Shapiro, M.D.*
900 East Thirtieth St., Suite 303
Austin 78705
(Treats patients up to age 21)

Scoliosis Associates
The Methodist Hospital
6550 Fannin
Houston 77030

Texas Scottish Rite Hospital
2222 Welborn St.
Dallas 75219
(Treats patients up to age 18)

The Center for Orthopaedic
    Surgery
c/o Highland University Medical
    Center
2424 50th St.
Lubbock 79412

The Orthopaedic Center
17270 Red Oak
Houston 77090

University of Texas Medical
    Branch
Pediatric Scoliosis Clinic
Child Health Center
Galveston 77550-2776
(Treats patients up to age 20)

W. B. Carrell Memorial Clinic,
    Assoc.
2909 Lemmon Ave.
Dallas 75204

Ira M. Yount, M.D., P.A.*
4499 Medical Dr., Suite 120
San Antonio 78229

Utah

Intermountain Clinic
350 South Seventh East
Salt Lake City 84102

Orthopedic Surgery Clinic
University of Utah Medical
    Center
50 North Medical Dr.
Salt Lake City 84132

Primary Children's Hospital
Salt Lake City 84102

Vermont

Medical Centre Hospital of
    Vermont
Burlington 05405

Spine Institute of New England
2 Hurricane Lane
P.O. Box 1043
Williston 05495

Virginia

Abingdon Orthopedic
  Associates, P.C.
300 East Valley St.
Abingdon 24210
(Treats patients up to age 21)

Arlington Orthopedic
  Associates, P.C.
300 East Valley St.
Arlington 24210

Children's Hospital
2924 Brook Rd.
Richmond 23220

Children's National Medical
  Center
Satellite Office
3299 Woodburn Rd.
Annandale 22003
(Treats patients up to age 18)

Fairfax Hospital
3300 Gallows Rd.
Falls Church 22046

Kluge Children's Rehabilitation
  Center
2270 Ivy Road
Charlottesville 22901

C. Michael Reing, M.D., P.C.*
3301 Woodbarn Rd.
Annandale 22004

Richmond Memorial Hospital
1300 Westwood Ave.
Richmond 23227

Richmond Orthopaedic Clinic,
  Ltd.
1400 Westwood Ave., Suite 204
Richmond 23227

The Children's Specialty Services
109 Governor St.
Richmond 23219
(Treats patients up to age 21)

Washington

Mary Bridge Children's Hospital
  and Health Center
311 South L Street
Tacoma 98405
(Treats children of all ages)

Childrens' Hospital & Medical
  Center
4800 Sand Point Way
Seattle 98105

Drs. Hurley, Lester, Osebold,
  Thompson & Jabszenski*
South 820 McClellan St., Room
  226
Spokane 99204

Northwest Spine Surgeons
4540 Sand Point Way N.E.,
  Room 140
Seattle 98105

Orthopedics International
1600 East Jefferson St., Room
  400
Seattle 98122

Orthopaedic Physicians, Inc.
1229 Madison St., Suite 1600
Seattle 98104

Swedish Hospital Medical Center
747 Summit Ave.
Seattle 98104

Seattle Orthopedic Clinic
801 Broadway
Seattle 98122

Shriners Hospital
North 820 Summit Blvd.
Spokane 99201

St. Luke's Memorial Hospital
South 711 Cowley
Spokane 99202

West Virginia

Charleston Scoliosis Clinic
Department of Handicapped
 Children
1116 Quarrier St.
Charleston 25301

Michael O. Fidler, M.D.*
3100 MacCorkle Ave., S.E.
Charleston 25304

Wisconsin

Blount Orthopaedic Clinic
625 East St. Paul Ave.
Milwaukee 53202

Children's Hospital
9000 West Wisconsin Ave.
Milwaukee 53226

Columbia Hospital
2025 East Newport Ave.
Milwaukee 53211

Drs. Flatley, Kubley,
 Langenkamp, and Benson*
2040 West Wisconsin Ave.
Milwaukee 53233

LaSalle Clinic
411 Lincoln St.
Neenah 54956

Madison General Hospital
202 South Park
Madison 53715

Madison Orthopaedics-
 Physicians Plus
20 South Park, Suite 455
Madison 53715

Orthopedic Associates of
 Milwaukee, S.C.
2350 West Villard Ave., Suite 111
Milwaukee 53209

St. Francis Hospital
3237 South Sixteenth St.
Milwaukee 53215

Theda Clark Regional Medical
 Center
Neenah 54956

University of Wisconsin
 Hospital and Clinics
600 Highland Ave.
Madison 53792

Bibliography

Allen, Ben L. "Segmental Instrumentation of the Spine—Indications, Results and Complications," in *Management of Spinal Deformities*, eds. Robert A. Dickson and David S. Bradford. London: Butterworth's International Medical Reviews, 1984.

Allen, Ben L., and Ron L. Ferguson. "The Galveston Technique for L Rod Instrumentation of the Scoliotic Spine," *Spine*, 7:3, 1982.

Barrack, Robert L., Marilynn P. Wyatt, Thomas S. Whitecloud III, Stephen W. Burke, John M. Roberts, and Mark R. Brinker. "Vibratory Hypersensitivity in Idiopathic Scoliosis," paper presented at the American Association of Orthopaedic Surgeons Convention in New Orleans, 1985.

Betz, Randall R., William P. Bunnell, Elizabeth Lambrecht-Mulier, and G. Dean MacEwen. "Scoliosis and Pregnancy, *The Journal of Bone and Joint Surgery*, Jan. 1987.

Blount, Walter P. "The Nonoperative Management of Scoliosis," *ONA Journal*, June 1976.

Borkovec, Thomas D., Lenore Wilkinson, Rowland Folensbee, and Caryn Lerman. "Stimulus Control Applications to the Treatment of Worry," *Behavioral Research Therapy*, 23:3, 1983.

Brickley-Parsons, Diane, and Melvin J. Glimcher. "Is the Chemistry of Collagen in Intervertebral Discs an Expression of Wolff's Law?" *Spine*, 9:2, 1984.

Bradford, David S. "New Spine Fixation Implant System Provides Encouraging Results." *Scoli News*. Minneapolis: Fairview Hospital, Fall 1985.

Bradford, David S., Katherine M. Cooper, and Theodore Oegema, Jr. "Chymopapain, Chemonucleolysis, and Nuclear Pulposus Regeneration," *Journal of Bone and Joint Surgery*, December 1983.

Bradford, David S., John E. Lonstein, John H. Moe, James W. Ogilvie, and Robert B. Winter. *Moe's Textbook of Scoliosis and Other Spinal Deformities*, 2nd ed. Philadelphia: W. B. Saunders, 1986.

Brown, John C., Jens Axelgaard, and David C. Howson. "Multicenter Trial of a Noninvasive Stimulation Method for Idiopathic Scoliosis," *Spine*, 9:4, 1984.

Bunch, Wilton H., and Victoria Dvonch. "Bracing for Idiopathic Scoliosis: Current Concepts," in *Management of Spinal Deformities*, eds. Robert A. Dickson and David S. Bradford. London: Butterworth's International Medical Reviews, 1984.

Bunnell, William P. "Orthotic Treatment of Spinal Deformity," in *The Pediatric Spine*, eds. David S. Bradford and Robert H. Hensinger. New York: Thieme, 1985.

———— "An Objective Criterion for Scoliosis Screening," *Journal of Bone and Joint Surgery*, December 1984.

Byers, Peter H. "Genetic Disorders of Connective Tissue Metabolism and Their Relation to Idiopathic Scoliosis," in *Pathogenesis of Idiopathic Scoliosis*, ed. Rae R. Jacobs. Chicago: Scoliosis Research Society, 1984.

Dienhart, Paul. "Straightened Back, Strengthened Character," *Health Sciences*, Summer 1983.

Drummond, Denis J. "The Natural History of Spine Deformity," in *The Pediatric Spine*, eds. David S. Bradford and Robert H. Hensinger. New York: Thieme, 1985.

Dunn, Harold K. "Spinal Biomechanics," in *The Pediatric Spine*, eds. David S. Bradford and Robert H. Hensinger. New York: Thieme, 1985.

Gillespie, Robert. "Juvenile and Adolescent Idiopathic Scoliosis," in *The Pediatric Spine*, eds. David S. Bradford and Robert Hensinger. New York: Thieme, 1985.

Greve, Carl, Eric Trachtenberg, William Opsahl, Ursula Abbott, and Robert Rucher. "Diet as an External Factor in the Expression of Scoliosis in a Line of Susceptible Chickens," *Journal of Nutrition*, volume 117, 1986.

Hall, John E. "Congenital Scoliosis," in *The Pediatric Spine*, eds. David S. Bradford and Robert Hensinger. New York: Thieme, 1985.

Herman, Richard M. "Postural and Ocular Motor Control in Patients with Idiopathic Scoliosis," in *Pathogenesis of Idiopathic Scoliosis*, ed. Rae R. Jacobs. Chicago: Scoliosis Research Society, 1984.

Herman, Richard M., James Mixon, Anne Fischer, Ruth Maulucci, and Joseph Stuyck. "Idopathic Scoliosis and the Central Nervous System: A Motor Control Problem," *Spine*, 10:1, 1985.

Herring, John A., and Dennis R. Wenger. "Segmental Spinal Instrumentation," *Spine*, 7:3, 1982.

Keim, Hugo A. *The Adolescent Spine*. New York: Springer-Verlag, 1982.

———— "Scoliosis Can Progress in the Adult," *Orthopaedic Review*, February 1974.

Koepfler, James W. "Moiré Topography in Medicine," *Journal of Biological Photography,* January 1983.

Lahde, Ruth Ellen. "Luque Rod Instrumentation," *AORN Journal,* July 1983.

Lonstein, John E., and Martin Carlson. "The Prediction of Curve Progression in Untreated Scoliosis During Growth," *Journal of Bone and Joint Surgery,* September 1984.

Luque, Eduardo. "The Luque System," in *The Pediatric Spine,* eds. David S. Bradford and Robert Hensinger. New York: Thieme, 1985.

Marchetti, Piere Giorgio. "Harrington Rods," in *The Pediatric Spine,* eds. David S. Bradford and Robert Hensinger. New York: Thieme, 1985.

Mayfield, Jack K. "Biomechanics of Spinal Deformities," in *Management of Spinal Deformities.* London: Butterworth's International Medical Reviews, 1984.

McMaster, Michael J. "Infantile Idiopathic Scoliosis," in *The Pediatric Spine,* eds. David S. Bradford and Robert Hensinger. New York: Thieme, 1985.

Moe, John H., Robert B. Winter, David S. Bradford, and John E. Lonstein. *Scoliosis and Other Spinal Deformities.* Philadelphia: W. B. Saunders, 1978.

Nachemson, Alf. "Future Research in Scoliosis: Possible Neuromuscular Causes," in *Pathogenesis of Idiopathic Scoliosis,* ed. Rae R. Jacobs. Chicago: Scoliosis Research Society, 1984.

Oegema, Theodore R., David S. Bradford, Katherine M. Cooper, and Robert E. Hunter. "Comparison of the Biochemistry of Proteoglycans Isolated from Normal, Idiopathic Scoliotic and Cerebral Palsy Spines," *Spine,* 8:4, 1983.

Opsahl, William, Ursula Abbott, Christina Kenney, and Robert Rucker. "Scoliosis in Chickens: Responsiveness of Severity and Incidence to Dietary Copper," *Science,* July 27, 1984.

O'Rahilly, Ronan, and Daniel R. Benson. "The Development of the Vertebral Column," in *The Pediatric Spine,* eds. David S. Bradford and Robert Hensinger. New York: Thieme, 1985.

Pratt, William B., James B. Schader, and William G. Phippen. "Elevation of Hair Copper in Idiopathic Scoliosis," *Spine,* 9:5, 1984.

Rucker, Robert, William Opsahl, Ursula Abbott, Carl Greve, Christina Kenney, and Robert Stern. "Scoliosis in Chickens: A Model for the Inherited Form of Adolescent Scoliosis," *American Journal of Pathology,* June 1986.

Sahlstrand, Tage, and Bjørn Petruson. "A Study of Labyrinthine Function in Patients with Adolescent Idiopathic Scoliosis," *Acta Orthopaedica Scandinavica,* Vol. 50, 1979.

Schommer, Nancy. "Standing Straight," *Discover,* December 1984.

Schultz, Albert B. "Biomechanical Factors in the Progression of Idiopathic Scoliosis," *Annals of Biomedical Engineering,* Vol. 12, 1984.

Stillings, Dennis. "A Survey of the History of Electrical Stimulation for Pain to 1900," *Medical Instrumentation*, November-December 1975.

Tredwell, Stephan J. "A Review of Possible Neuromuscular Causes," in *Pathogenesis of Idiopathic Scoliosis*. Chicago: Scoliosis Research Society, 1984.

Willner, Stig. "A Comprehensive Study of Efficiency of Different Types of School Screening for Scoliosis," *Acta Orthopaedica Scandinavica*, October 1982.

———— "The Interrelationship of Growth, Height and Skeletal Maturity in Scoliosis," in *Pathogenesis of Idiopathic Scoliosis*. Chicago: Scoliosis Research Society, 1984.

Wilson, John F. "Behavioral Preparation for Surgery: Benefit or Harm?" *Journal of Behavioral Medicine*, 4:1, 1981.

Winter, Robert B. "Adolescent Idiopathic Scoliosis," *New England Journal of Medicine*, May 22, 1986.

Yamada, Kengo, Hiroshi Yamamoto, Yukio Nakagawa, Akitsugu Tezuka, Taishi Tamura, and Shoji Kawata. "Etiology of Idiopathic Scoliosis," *Clinical Orthopedics and Related Research*, April 1984.

Yamamoto, Hiroshi. "A Postural Dysequilibrium as an Etiological Factor in Idiopathic Scoliosis," in *Pathogenesis of Idiopathic Scoliosis*. Chicago: Scoliosis Research Society, 1984.

Index